JUNGIAN ANALYSIS

POST MORTEM DEI

JUNGIAN ANALYSIS

POST MORTEM DEI

Greg Mogenson

DUSK OWL BOOKS
London, Ontario, Canada

A title in the monograph series of
The International Society for Psychology as the Discipline of Interiority, Vol. 6

Published by
Dusk Owl Books
London, Ontario, Canada

Cover design and typesetting by
Michael Mendis

ISBN 978-1-9992266-5-7

CONTENTS

Acknowledgments

This essay was first published in *Spring: A Journal of Archetype and Culture*, Vol. 84, Fall, 2010, pages 207-270. Although originally intended as a response to an article by Wolfgang Giegerich, I offer it here in a slightly adapted version to be read on its own as a stand-alone piece. For more information about Giegerich's article and the collegial exchange that took place in that issue of *Spring*, the reader is directed to the "Guest Editor's Introduction" that I wrote for that occasion (pp. 1-10). It is republished here as an Appendix to this book.

SOURCES AND ABBREVIATIONS

The following abbreviations have been used for frequently cited sources:

CEP: Wolfgang Giegerich, *The Collected English Papers of Wolfgang Giegerich*, 6 vols., New Orleans: Spring Journal Books, 2005-2013. Cited by volume and page number. All volumes have been republished since 2020 by Routledge. Giegerich's article "God Must Not Die! C.G. Jung's Thesis of the One-Sidedness of Christianity" appears in *CEP*, Vol. VI, Chapter IV.

CW: Carl Gustav Jung, *Collected Works*, 20 vols. Herbert Read, Michael Fordham, Gerhard Adler and William McGuire, eds., R. F. C. Hull, trans., Princeton: Princeton University Press, 1957-1979. Cited by volume and paragraph number.

MDR: C. G. Jung, *Memories, Dreams, Reflections*. Rev. ed., Aniela Jaffé. Trans. Richard and Clara Winston. New York: Vintage Books, 1989, cited by page number.

Letters: C. G. Jung, *Letters*. 2 vols. Ed. Gerhard Adler. Bollingen Series XCV: 2. Princeton: Princeton University Press, 1975.

Spring: *Spring: A Journal of Archetype and Culture*, New Orleans: Spring Journal Books. Cited by volume number, in some cases by year.

Part One

It is for your own good that I am going. Because unless I go the Paraclete will not come to you; but if I do go, I will send him to you.

John 16:7

The God-Question

It has sometimes happened in the course of an analysis that a patient has asked me if I believe in God. Recalling such occasions, the rule of these has been: they have always occurred in what would have seemed the most unlikely of cases. That *this* patient would ask of me *that* question, why, I would have never expected it. During the whole of our previous work together no indication of religious interests, let alone of any tendency to *think* in religious categories, had ever been communicated. On the contrary, session after session, week in and week out, talk about some private misery stubbornly held sway. The troubled marriage, the envied co-worker, the latest imposition or affront: no matter how thoroughly these topics were discussed, there was always more to say about them—transcendence be damned. Or so it seemed, until one day the question was put to me: "Do you believe in God?"

Now it might be thought, given the well-known response of C. G. Jung to the same question, that an affirmative answer would come readily to the lips of any subsequent member of his guild. I allude here to the interview that the BBC conducted with Jung in 1959 for its television series "Face to Face." Asked if he believed in God, the 85-year-old psychologist balked at first at the word "believe." God for him was no matter of belief. As he famously stated at the time, "I *know*. I don't need to believe. I know."[1]

A precious statement, this. Preserved on film, it is a part of our spiritual heritage. And yet, if the interview were to be re-broadcast today, some Grand Inquisitor of Correctness would require a disclaimer to be added: "The opinions expressed in this programme do not necessarily reflect the theory and practice of contemporary Jungian analysis."

The issue here is an ethical one. As analysts we are concerned about the deleterious effects of imposing our beliefs upon our patients. For what a doubtful enterprise analysis would be if our patients had to become like us, believing as we do, to become authenticated. But this said, there has also been a tradition within analytical psychology of valuing candour on the part of the analyst. In a lecture series that he gave at the Tavistock Clinic in 1935 Jung spoke of this to an audience largely made up of Freudian colleagues: "I put my patients in front of me and talk to them as one natural human being to another, and I expose myself completely and react with no restriction" (*CW* 18 § 319). Setting this technical recommendation alongside his other statement about knowing God, we may be prompted to ask: if it is not a matter of belief, but of knowledge, is a reply by the analyst to the God-question *de rigueur* after all?

Jung, evidently, thought that it was. In yet another interview given in his old age, knowledge based upon religious experience was authoritatively declared by him to be the very touchstone of the analytic process:

> Without knowing it man is always concerned with God. What some people call instinct or intuition is nothing other than God. God is that voice inside us which tells us what to do and what not to do. In other words, our conscience. ... I make my patients understand that all the things which happen to them against their will are a superior force. They can call it God or devil, and that doesn't matter to me, as long as they realize that it is a superior force. God is nothing more than that superior force in our life. You can experience God every day.[2]

---

[1] BBC Television, "Face to Face," broadcast October 22, 1959. In W. McGuire & R.F.C. Hull, eds., *C. G. Jung Speaking: Interviews and Encounters* (Princeton: Princeton University Press, 1977), p. 428.

[2] McGuire & Hull, eds., *C.G. Jung Speaking*, pp. 249-250.

This statement, it is important to stress, was not intended as a theological assertion. It concerned, rather, Jung's psychological vision and analytic stance. When conveying his position as a psychologist with respect to the reality of the psyche, Jung drew upon divine epithets. Psychological reality, in his view, was a matter of what he called "immanent-transcendental" experience (*CW* 18 § 1505). Arising immanently out of inner subjective depths, it could be called transcendent at the same time inasmuch as our experiences happen to us.[3] And it was from this, let us call it the "objective" or even "divine" character of psychic reality, that Jung's use of "God" and "the unconscious" as synonymous terms stemmed. Just as the unconscious can be revelatory, so God, according to Jung, is "one of the most certain and immediate experiences," "as plain as a brick that falls on your head …" (*MDR*, p. 62).

The great psychologist could not have been more adamant. And yet, to the careful reader such statements were by no means as unequivocal as they at first may have seemed. For even after repeated readings one could still wonder if the God that Jung spoke about in such tangible and concrete terms was of the same order of reality as the God that believers relate to through their faith. And so, wanting to know where he really stood many attempted to hold his feet to the fire on this question. But what had once been a fire to test heretics had waned in the meantime to the mere glow of a fading coal. Or was this coal, even as it faded, the ember of a new consciousness?

Psychologizing God

"I have been asked so often whether I believe in the existence of God," wrote Jung in *Answer to Job*, "that I am somewhat concerned lest I be taken for an adherent of 'psychologism.' What

---

[3] I allude here to the following passage of Jung's: "The ego stands to the self as the moved to the mover, or as object to subject, because the determining factors which radiate out from the self surround the ego on all sides and are therefore supraordinate to it. The self, like the unconscious, is an *a priori* existent out of which the ego evolves. … *It is not I who create myself, rather I happen to myself*." (*CW* 11 § 391, italics mine)

most people overlook or seem unable to understand is the fact that I regard the psyche as *real.* … God is an obvious psychic and non-physical fact, i.e., a fact that can be established psychically but not physically" (*CW* 11 § 751).

The knowledge that Jung claimed with respect to God had to do with what could be known empirically about the soul as a psychologist. And if, as he put it, he did not need to believe because he knew, this knowing was based upon the empirical study of human ideas and human beliefs, that is, upon the phenomenology of religious experience both personal and communal.

As for his use of "God" and "the unconscious" as synonymous terms and his reference to "inner, transcendental experience" (*CW* 10 § 511), what Jung had in mind with these gestures and associations is evident from a passage from the 2nd century gnostic writer, Monoïmos, that he quoted in *Aion*:

> Seek him from out thyself, and learn who it is that taketh possession of everything in thee, saying: *my* god, *my* spirit, *my* understanding, *my* soul, *my* body; and learn whence is sorrow and joy, and love and hate, and waking though one would not, and sleeping though one would not, and getting angry though one would not, and falling in love though one would not. And if thou shouldst closely investigate these things, thou wilt find Him in thyself, the One and the Many, like to that little point … for it is in thee that he hath his origin and his deliverance. (Cited in *CW* 9, ii § 347)

Just as the ancient author of this passage directs the seeker after God to the kinds of experiences that the modern psychoanalyst identifies with the unconscious, so Jung, many centuries later, advised his analysands to seek after the unconscious in the name of God.[4]

---

[4] Justifying his identification of God and the unconscious Jung resorts to an epistemological style of argument: "It is only through the psyche that we can establish that God acts upon us, but we are unable to distinguish whether these actions emanate from God or from the unconscious. We cannot tell whether God and the unconscious are two different entities. Both are border-line concepts for transcendental contents. But empirically it can be established, with a sufficient degree of probability, that there is in the unconscious an archetype of

But what of the "how" and the "when," the "why" and the "wherefore" of using now one, now the other, of these interchangeable terms? In a discussion of this topic Jung explained that as a scientist and psychological theorist he "prefer[ed] the term 'the unconscious'" because it was "coined for scientific purposes" and was, thus, "better suited to dispassionate observation" than were its mythological equivalents. It was a different matter, however, when it came to his psychotherapeutic work. In that context his preference was to speak of "'mana,' 'daimon,' and 'God'" as he felt that these terms facilitated an altogether more vivid engagement with the psychic process.

> … for certain purposes … belief is far more useful and effective than a scientific concept. The great advantage of the concepts "daimon" and "God" lies in making possible a much better objectification of the *vis-à-vis*, namely, a *personification* of it. Their emotional quality confers life and effectuality upon them. Hate and love, fear and reverence, enter the scene of the confrontation and raise it to a drama. What has merely been "displayed" becomes "acted." The whole man is challenged and enters the fray with his total reality. Only then can he become whole and only then can "God be born," that is, enter into human reality and associate with man in the form of "man." By this act of incarnation man—that is, his ego—is inwardly replaced by "God," and God becomes outwardly man, in keeping with the saying of Jesus: "Who sees me, sees the Father." (*MDR*, p. 337)

---

wholeness which manifests itself spontaneously in dreams, etc., and a tendency, independent of the conscious will, to relate other archetypes to this centre. Consequently, it does not seem improbable that the archetype of wholeness occupies as such a central position which approximates it to the God-image. … These facts make possible a certain qualification of our above thesis concerning the indistinguishableness of God and the unconscious. Strictly speaking, the God-image does not coincide with the unconscious as such, but with a special content of it, namely the archetype of the self. It is this archetype from which we can no longer distinguish the God-image empirically." (*CW* 11 § 757)

Psychology, a Religion?

From the passages that I have quoted it is not surprising that Jung should have had to again and again respond to the question of whether analytical psychology is a religion. His answer, of course, was always to reject this admittedly understandable impression. Analytical psychology, he said, is not a religion, nor he a religious leader. His disclaimers, however, did little to settle the controversies that his playing so fast and loose with the God-concept stirred up.

In a 1922 letter to Freud, for example, an early defector from Jung's circle, the Protestant minister and lay-analyst Oskar Pfister, declared himself "finished with the Jungian manner":

> Those high-falutin interpretations which proclaim every kind of muck to be spiritual jam of a high order and try to smuggle a minor Apollo or Christ into every corked-up little mind simply will not do. It is Hegelianism transferred to psychology; everything that is must be reasonable. If only that theory were true![1]

And then, toward the end of his life and career, there was the rather bitter exchange between Jung and Martin Buber. Basing himself upon a thorough reading of Jung's texts, the great Jewish philosopher had charged Jung with bringing about an "eclipse of God" through his having substituted for the concept of an externally existing deity a false "religion of pure psychic immanence."[2] Jung, of course, defended himself manfully on his side of this public exchange. Not one to eat his words, he did find, however, that he had to chew over them more carefully in his subsequent response and in the many letters to correspondents that followed in the aftermath of this and the "Face to Face" interview which was broadcast some years later.

---

[1] Sigmund Freud & Oskar Pfister, *Psychoanalysis and Faith: The Letters of Sigmund Freud and Oskar Pfister* (London: Hogarth Press and the Institute of Psycho-Analysis, 1963), pp. 86-87.

[2] Martin Buber, *Eclipse of God: Studies in the Relation between Religion and Philosophy* (New York: Harper & Row, 1952), p. 84.

"What I have described is a psychic factor only," he wrote in his "Reply to Buber,"

> but one which exerts a considerable influence on the conscious mind. Thanks to its autonomy, it forms the counterposition to the subjective ego because it is a piece of the *objective psyche*. It can therefore be designated as a "Thou." For me its reality is amply attested by the truly diabolical deeds of our time: the six million murdered Jews, the uncounted victims of the slave labour camps in Russia, as well as the invention of the atom bomb, to name but a few examples of the darker side. But I have also seen the other side which can be expressed by the words beauty, goodness, wisdom, grace. These experiences of the depths and heights of human nature justify the metaphorical use of the term "daimon." (*CW* 18 § 1505)

We had just heard in the section above this one Jung's argument for the *therapeutic* advantages of using mythological terms and speaking the language of belief. Now, in defence of his frequent references to God *in his scientific writings*, he clarifies that what he refers to in this way "is a psychic factor only," but one that justifies "the metaphorical use" of the terms daimon and God. It might be wondered if Jung is drawing in his horns a little here. What has happened to the God that he did not believe in, but knew? While continuing to make reference to God, Jung now owns up to this as being a *façon de parler* that is useful in psychotherapy, "a psychic factor only," a metaphor.

Quite a comedown, this rejoinder! Jung, evidently, had become aware of the vainglorious tenor of his claims with respect to God and seeking to redress this hastened to express himself in a more psychologically circumspect manner. Such, at any rate, is the impression that comes across from a reply that he penned to a correspondent who had written to him following the "Face to Face" interview:

> Mr. Freeman [the BBC interviewer] in his characteristic manner fired the question you allude to at me in a somewhat surprising way, so that I was perplexed and had to say the next thing which came into my mind. As soon as the answer had left the "edge of my teeth" I knew I had said something controversial, puzzling,

> or even ambiguous. I was therefore just waiting for letters like yours. Mind you, I didn't say, "there is a God," I said: "I don't need to believe in God, I *know*." Which does not mean: I do know a certain God (Zeus, Yahweh, Allah, the Trinitarian God, etc.) but rather: I do know that I am obviously confronted with a factor unknown in itself and which I call "God" in *consensu omnium (quod semper, quod ubique, quod ab omnibus creditur)*. (*Letters* 2, p. 525, to M. Leonard, 5 December 1959)

In this passage Jung demurs somewhat with respect to his controversial statement about knowing God. Perplexed by the abruptness of the interviewer's question, he had answered with the first thing that came into his mind. His answer, thus, had not been a well-considered one. It had had more the character of a reaction to one of the stimulus words that he used to detect complexes with in the word association experiments of his early days.[3] But while this was certainly true on this particular occasion, what are we to

---

[3] Further to this point, it is worth noting that Jung's whole concept of God seems to be redolent of his word association experiment research and his concept of the complex. In the lines immediately following those we are discussing here, he continues: "I remember Him, I evoke Him, whenever I use His name, overcome by anger or by fear, whenever I involuntarily say: 'Oh God.' That happens when I meet somebody or something stronger than myself. It is an apt name given to all overpowering emotions in my own psychic system, subduing my conscious will and usurping control over myself. This is the name by which I designate all things which cross my wilful path violently and recklessly, all things which upset my subjective views, plans, and intentions and change the course of my life for better or worse" (*Letters* 2, p. 525, to M. Leonard, 5 December 1959). Likewise in his 1906 article, "The Psychopathological Significance of the Association Experiment," Jung states that "The occurrences of everyday life are nothing but association experiments on a major scale; the things outside us are the stimulus-words to which we react …" (*CW* 2 § 895). It could be argued from this basis that Jung's concept of God was overdetermined and undermined by his concept of the complex. While it may be possible to speak of a God-complex, it will hardly do to approach the notion or concept of God as if it were a complex. Although in this essay we are interested, not in the God-complex, but in the God-concept, Jung, doubtless, had such a complex. Aniela Jaffé writes of the ten-year-old Jung's overhearing his pastor father's pathetic prayers imploring God to help him to believe as constituting a childhood trauma. His later distinction between believing and knowing may be a part of his answer to his father's plight. Aniela Jaffé, *Was C. G. Jung A Mystic? And Other Essays* (Einsiedeln: Daimon Verlag, 1989), p. 89.

make of the other times when Jung said the same thing in a more considered manner?

An interview given in 1955 that Jung *was* able to read and approve prior to its publication in the *London Daily Mail* concluded with these words: "All that I have learned has led me step by step to an unshakable conviction of the existence of God. I only believe in what I know. And that eliminates believing. Therefore I do not take His existence on belief—I *know* that he exists."[4] Again, as in the "Face to Face" interview, Jung speaks most adamantly. On this occasion, however, he does not rest content with merely drawing his psychological distinction between believing and knowing, or confine himself to a psychic factor only; on top of this he affirms the *existence* of God!

What is going on here? In Jung's usual phenomenological/ empirical sense of knowing, knowing God means fathoming the meaning of any God-image, even if it were to be the image or idea of the death of God. But now he makes an ontological claim. He refers to the *existence* of God; he says, "I *know* that he exists."

It would seem that with these words Jung's position with respect to a really existing deity is stated in no uncertain terms and that theists everywhere can simply claim him as one of their own. This, however, is a mistaken impression arising, I believe, from the assumption that the meaning of his statement is the same as it would be if it were spoken from someone else's mouth. What Jung actually has in mind is a very different matter. And to get at this we must be able to square his statement about having been "led to an unshakable conviction of the existence of God" with the many others that fly in the face of it, such as the warning he issued on another occasion: "It would be a regrettable mistake if anybody should take my observations as a kind of proof of the existence of God. They prove only the existence of an archetypal God-image, which to my mind is the most we can assert about God psychologically" (*CW* 11 § 102; cf., *CW* 14 § 781).

No easy feat, the squaring of this circle. Reading now the one, now the other of Jung's statements, we may feel that we have come across an inconsistency or contradiction, even. But while this may

[4] McGuire & Hull, eds., *C. G. Jung Speaking*, p. 251.

be so, there is reason for the reader to persevere. Inconsistency and contradiction, after all, are not only the hallmarks of misconception and error; they can also herald the appearance of new truth. And this, arguably, was the case with Jung. Taken together, his inconsistent and contradicting statements were the avowal of a new God-term (though it is perhaps no longer appropriate to call it that): the *coincidentia oppositorum* of *Psychology itself* in the highest determination of Jung's conception of it.[5]

Reversing the Relation

In the previous pages a small, but representative sample of the kinds of statements that Jung made when queried about his religious beliefs has been examined. And following upon this we have just now ventured the thesis that as a psychologist Jung had had to grapple with such questions, not because his analytical psychology was a religion, but because psychology in his sense is the successor to religion. Extending this a bit, it could also be said that Jung was not first a psychologist who then transgressed the boundaries of his profession to take positions on theological questions; rather, it was the other way around: it was his tackling of the God question again and again that produced his sense of the psychological as its result.

Numerous texts come to mind in support of this contention. I will here mention only two, from "The Archetypes of the Collective Unconscious." In answer to the question—"Why is psychology the youngest of the empirical sciences? Why have we not long since discovered the unconscious and raised up its treasure-house of eternal images?"—Jung replies: "Simply because we [formerly had] had a religious formula for everything psychic—and one that is far more beautiful and comprehensive than immediate experience" (*CW* 9, i § 11). Developing this point

[5] Of course, it is true: many of Jung's inconsistencies can be explained by his having expressed himself in different ways to different audiences. This, however, does not relieve us of the challenge of reading his various statements in the light of one another. Jung needed a wide and disparate audience in order to say what he had to say. Each statement, then, may be considered to be a mediating, differentiating, individuating moment of a single position or concept.

further in a later passage he then explains that an "unparalleled impoverishment of [religious] symbolism" was what opened the way for our "rediscovery of the gods as psychic factors, that is, as archetypes of the unconscious":

> Since the stars have fallen from heaven and our highest symbols have paled, a secret life holds sway in the unconscious. That is why we have a psychology today, and why we speak of the unconscious. All this would be quite superfluous in an age or culture that possessed symbols. Symbols are spirit from above, and under those conditions the spirit is above too. Therefore it would be a foolish and senseless undertaking for such people to wish to experience or investigate an unconscious that contains nothing but the silent, undisturbed sway of nature. Our unconscious, on the other hand, hides living water, spirit that has become nature, and that is why it is disturbed. (*CW* 9, i § 50)

The provenance of psychology, according to these passages of Jung's, resides in the decline of the religions that preceded it. Having encountered one another in the various ways that modernity made possible, the World's religions contradicted or at least relativized one another. No longer could any one of them simply take the universality of its symbols for granted. Comparison and doubt had entered the picture. And, yet, the upshot of this mutually negating witness yielded an affirmative result. As what the various religions held in common became discernable, consciousness advanced to a higher level of complexity than it had had within the single faiths that it pushed off from in this way. This, at least, has been the case with Jung's psychology, which, by its own account, has given the truths of the religions a new form as what he called the archetypes of the collective unconscious.

But what about Christianity? While Jung was certainly interested in what could be learned about the psyche from the study of comparative religion, Christianity held a special significance for him as the most immediate precursor of modern psychology generally and of his analytical psychology in particular. Why, it could even be argued that his wider interest in comparative religion was redolent of a Christian story. Guided by Christ's star, the Magi from the East travelled from distant lands to Bethlehem to bestow their gifts upon the infant Jesus. Likewise, with his culture-transcending, religion-sublating concept of the collective unconscious, Jung followed a sunken version of that same star to the scene of that most ecumenical of all nativities, the nativity of psychology.[1]

Now my reference here is to a "sunken" star because in Jung's view it is "as the intensity of the Christian ideas begins to *fade*, [that] a recrudescence of individual symbol-formation may be expected" (*CW* 8 § 92, italics mine). No longer insulated from the actuality of our life's truth by the cultural mediation that the Christian faith had provided during the course of its flourishing, the individual is subjected to a veritable onslaught of immediate experiences, as the stigmata of his symptomatic suffering attest. Drawing upon Christian ideas, Jung regarded this experience, this suffering, to be constituted by a post-Christian outpouring of the Holy Spirit upon the many. Overflowing themselves, the symbols of Christianity became metaphors, symptoms, and psychological terms, even.

Examples abound. With regard to work with patients in the consulting room Jung declared: "Analysis should release an experience that grips us or falls upon us as from above, an experience that has substance and body such as those things which occurred to the ancients. If I were going to symbolize it I would choose the Annunciation."[2] Continuing the analogy, he writes on other occasions of the incarnate Christ as a model of the human individuation process: "The drama of the archetypal life of Christ describes in symbolic images the events in the conscious life—as well as in the life that transcends consciousness—of a man who has been transformed by his higher destiny" (*CW* 11 § 223).[3] Another important reference is to Pentecost. Consistent with his view that psychology is itself a kind of myth inasmuch as its theories are underpinned by the same archetypes that underpinned

---

[1] For a fuller treatment of this topic see my *The Dove in the Consulting Room: Hysteria and the Anima in Bollas and Jung* (Hove & New York: Brunner-Routledge, 2003).

[2] C. G. Jung, *Notes of the Seminar Given in 1925*, W. McGuire, ed. (Princeton: Princeton University Press, 1989), p. 111.

[3] Cf.: "What happens in the life of Christ happens always and everywhere. In the Christian archetype all lives of this kind are prefigured." (*CW* 11 § 146)

religion, Jung avers that the "further development of myth might well begin with the outpouring of the Holy Spirit upon the apostles [at Pentecost], by which they were made into sons of God ..." (*MDR*, p. 333). And, of course, in this connection we should also mention Jesus' reference to the Paraclete. Speaking to the disciples at the Last Supper, Jesus assured them that it was good that he was going to his death, for only with his going away could his spiritual form come to dwell within them and be known to them (John 16:7). Carrying this reference of Jesus' to the Paraclete ("Advocate" or "Comforter") forward into psychology, Jung identifies the action of this figure with the spontaneous manifestation of the unconscious in the modern individual, i.e., with the aforementioned "recrudescence of individual symbol-formation" that arises with the decline of religious symbolism:

> Despite the fact that he is potentially redeemed, the Christian [we may also read here, the patient or analysand—G.M.] is given over to moral suffering, and in his suffering he needs the Comforter, the Paraclete. He cannot overcome the conflict on his own resources; after all, he didn't invent it. He has to rely on divine comfort and mediation, that is to say on the spontaneous revelation of the spirit, which does not obey man's will but comes and goes as *it* wills. The spirit is an autonomous psychic happening, a hush that follows the storm, a reconciling light in the darknesses of man's mind, secretly bringing order into the chaos of his soul. (*CW* 11 § 260)

A Sheepish Feeling

In the above reflections we have been discussing the spirit of analytical psychology in relation to responses that Jung gave when questioned about his belief in God. While doing so, however, the situation that we began with, in which *I* was the addressee of this question, has not been forgotten. This, on the contrary, has been with me all along. But as on those occasions, so now in these pages: thoughts and associations have flashed to mind just as they did during the long seconds that ticked by as my patients' questions hung in the air between us.

Of course, I know that I do not have to answer, not then and not now. And I suspect, moreover, that my patients may have already known that as an analyst I very likely would not. But there is pressure all the same. A question has been asked and an answer is expected. Ordinary human etiquette, if not the rules of analysis, places an onus upon me.

And yet, as obliging as I would like to be, a certain wariness prevails. This I suspect may have partly to do with the strife-ridden history that has long been associated with matters of religion. More blood has been spilled over disputes about God than over any other cause. Would what I might say suffice for the inquisition writ small that this moment has become? And then, on the heels of this reflection, I am subject to a sheepish feeling. I think to myself about how halting and complicated my answer has probably become, though it be to a question for which my career as a Jungian analyst had once seemed to provide of itself such a hearty and affirmative answer. But faithful to my training, if to nothing else, I return the question unanswered to its sender. For what good is *my* belief to my patient? And by the same token, what good is *Jung's* to me? If there is a God to be found he only exists through each one's finding their own. "No one besides you has your God,"[1] writes Jung in his *Red Book*.

Caveat Redemptor

But wait! Is this really enough? Batted back and forth like a shuttlecock or hot potato, has not the question we began with been short-changed in the interaction I have just described? The problem here is not with the idea of finding one's own. That's true enough, each one must find into their own. The issue, rather, is with whether "one's own" must have the form of God. Reviewing what I have written, I notice that my final reflection shows a theistic bias. Effacing what the question—Do you believe in God?—actually asks, the thoughts through which I released myself from having to answer simply assume (to say it with the words of

[1] C. G. Jung, *The Red Book: Liber Novus*, S. Shamdasani, ed. (New York & London, W. W. Norton & Company, 2009), p. 329.

the oracle that Jung inscribed above his doorway in Küsnacht) that "summoned or not summoned, the God will be there." The other option, i.e., that there could be a non-theistic, atheistic, or post-theistic answer, is not even considered. Perhaps, then, in light of this, and in the interest of restoring the larger sense of the question, its addressee should no longer be the analyst or patient, *but psychology itself*. The challenge of this, let us now call it *"the soul's" own question*, would then become (given analytical psychology's rootedness in a religious sensibility) to consider whether Jungian analysis is conceivable *in absentia dei*, or to anticipate a bit what is to come in Part Two and Three below, whether it is conceivable *post mortem dei*.

Part Two

> [We] should bend to the great task of reinterpreting all the Christian traditions … [and since] it is a question of truths which are anchored deep in the soul … the solution of this task must be possible.
>
> C. G. Jung, *Answer to Job* (*CW* 11 § 754)

"God Must Not Die!"—or Must He, Has He?

We now come to the article of Giegerich's to which the volume of *Spring Journal* in which the present essay first appeared was devoted.[1] In formulating a response to it, my interest will be to show its critical importance with respect to the problematic that has been outlined above in Part One.

Jung, as we have been discussing, regarded God to be the touchstone of what he meant by soul even as the religions generally "express[ed] the whole range of the psychic problem in mighty images" (*CW* 10 § 367). And further to this, his psychology of individuation and self was predicated upon his interpretation of Christianity. By attending to dreams and other immanently transcendental psychic phenomena, the analytic process, in his view, was to "*dream the myth onwards* and give it a modern dress" (*CW* 9, i § 271). Turning now to Giegerich's essay, the first thing to be noted is how aptly its title—"God Must Not Die!"—sums up the main thrust of this, let us call it Jung's theistic conception

[1] Wolfgang Giegerich, "God Must Not Die! C. G. Jung's Thesis of the One-Sidedness of Christianity," *Spring:* Vol. 84, pp. 11-71. Reprinted in *CEP*, vol. 4, pp. 165-242.

of psychology. Jung, as Giegerich has discussed elsewhere,[2] had wanted "a situation in which that thing [that had previously been mediated by Christian symbolism] becomes true once more ..." (*CW* 18 § 632). He had wanted, that is to say, that what he called "the symbolic life" should still be possible, even after the decline of collective symbolism. The realization of this want, however, was far from straightforward. Having become conscious of consciousness itself, modern man was divided by this awareness from what has been called the Age of Faith. Where formerly the existence of God had been an almost universal conviction, it had become possible, even fashionable in the 19th and 20th centuries to debate and question this. Jung, of course, knew where he stood on this matter. From childhood on he had regarded God to be one of the most certain of experiences (*MDR*, p. 62). As a mature psychologist and man of his times, however, he had also to reckon with the fact that consciousness had advanced to its current stage of development largely by negating God. And herein lay the tension in which his life's work was forged. Unable to go back as a believer to the symbolism of Christianity (since he "[knew] too much about it"), Jung sought instead to establish "a new form" to provide for the same needs (*CW* 18 § 632). This form, as we have already indicated, was the form of psychology, or to be more specific, of *the psychology of the unconscious.*

Simply put Jung's conception of the unconscious provided him with a counter-position to Nietzsche's atheism. The God whom Nietzsche had declared to be dead, and who had become less and less important in the conscious lives of Jung's contemporaries, was still a compelling reality according to Jung, along with a pantheon of other gods, in the realm of the unconscious.

Again, as we noted earlier, it was a case of falling stars, or as Fr. Victor White put it in his *God and the Unconscious*, of a "new disease of unconscious religion which becomes epidemic when man

---

[2] Wolfgang Giegerich, "The End of Meaning and the Birth of Man: An Essay about the State Reached in the History of Consciousness and an Analysis of C. G. Jung's Psychology Project," *Journal of Jungian Theory and Practice*, Vol. 6, No. 1, 2004, p. 38. Reprinted in *CEP* VI, p. 241,

is filched of his gods."[3] Finding support in analytical psychology for his ministry to an increasingly secular age, White, a Dominican priest who published under ecclesiastical *imprimatur*, cited Jung: "… whenever the Spirit of God is excluded from human consideration, an unconscious substitute takes its place." "The Gods have become diseases; not Zeus but the solar plexus now rules Olympus." And again, "When God is not recognized, selfish desires develop, and out of this selfishness comes illness."[4]

But is there another selfishness (and with it, another illness)? A selfishness that does not deny God or fail to recognize him, but that stubbornly insists upon him? In the essay under discussion, Giegerich argues that there is and offers Jung up as the prime example. The touchstone of his analysis consists of references of Jung's to God along with certain features of the latter's interpretation of Christianity. Jung, as Giegerich shows, so insists upon a psychology *with God* that he is prepared to don the mantle of a myth-maker to provide one. Railing against such things as the apparent cruelty of Yahweh to Job, the sacrifice of Christ as the behest of a loving Father, and the divine and semi-divine status of Jesus and Mary which he regards as casting the incarnation into doubt, Jung, in something of the manner of today's narrative therapies, supplies what Giegerich calls a "super-myth" wherein the unconscious and ethically inferior Jewish-Christian God becomes conscious and redeemed in the wholeness that individuals may achieve as the result of their individuation processes.

As Jungians, of course, we all know this story. Not only is God unconscious (in the sense of being irresponsible with respect to his dark side), Christianity is one-sided. Hallowed as being without sin, the canonical Jesus lacks completeness. The remedy for this, according to Jung, lies in the compensatory potential of the counter-tradition, specifically, in the legends that cropped up concerning the Antichrist. Just as the puerile Peter Pan had had to have his shadow sewn to his heel, so the spotless Christ must

---

[3] Victor White, *God and the Unconscious: An Encounter between Psychology and Religion* (London & Glasgow: Fontana Books, 1960), p. 43.

[4] These quotations from Jung are White's translations from the German. Their *Collected Works* equivalents are: *CW* 8 § 359, *CW* 13 § 54, and *CW* 13 § 55 respectively.

integrate Satan. And then there is the problem of the Trinity. Regarded by Jung as being incomplete, it, too, must be transformed through the inclusion of evil, for only by becoming four-fold in this manner is the wholeness of God adequately presented. This, however, cannot be achieved by God alone. It requires human help. And this is where the human individuation process, characterized by Jung as "life in God,"[5] comes in. Subject to ethical dilemmas that are not of his own making, the individual is the vessel, as it were, of the divine opposites that are operative in the back of these, contributing to their synthesis through the choices that he makes. And "that," writes Jung with "the myth of the necessary incarnation of God" in mind, "is the meaning of divine service, of the service which man can render to God, that light may emerge from the darkness, that the Creator may become conscious of His creation, and man conscious of himself. (*MDR*, p. 338)

Now it is important to remember that in propounding these ideas Jung made no attempt to limit himself to a "carefully considered exegesis that tries to be fair to every detail ..." (*CW* 11 § 561). On the contrary, inspired by what he called "the shattering emotion which the unvarnished spectacle of divine savagery and ruthlessness produces in us," he wrote as one who has pulled out all the stops (*ibid.*). Little wonder, then, that his interpretation of Christianity sounded in mighty organ blasts! Upon closer examination, however, the astute reader may doubt that Jung's thoughts on these matters are truly *interpretative* in character. Interpretation, after all, is not an anthem of stormy affects.[6] Its aim and purpose are simply to bring out the truth of the matter at hand, not to dream it along by imagining what should have been or could be.

But, of course, with respect to the psychology that bore his name, Jung enjoyed free rein. And if, as he once put it, he was glad

---

[5] "*Individuation is the life in God*, as mandala psychology clearly shows" (*CW* 18 § 1624).

[6] In a letter to Henry Corbin, Jung describes his coming to write *Answer to Job* as follows: "The book 'came to me' during the fever of an illness. It was as if accompanied by the great music of a Bach or a Handel .... I just had the feeling of listening to a great composition, or rather of being at a concert." 4 May, 1953, *Letters* 2, p. 116.

that he was Jung and not a Jungian, this may have been in part because his interpretations had the distinction of being Jungian just by virtue of the fact that *he* had announced them. For us who follow, however, it is not so easy. We have to ask, with a rigour that Jung often spared himself, if the interpretations that have come down to us from him are truly psychological in the fullest sense that he rightly gave to that term.

This, to be sure, is no small challenge. Jung was a great man, a psychologist of enormous stature. Amongst the generations of his followers there have been only a very few who have possessed the wherewithal, let alone the temerity, to challenge his views. Giegerich, to his credit, has long been one of these. Writing in what might be called a "*with* Jung, *against* Jung, *beyond* Jung spirit" he has for upwards of forty years been turning Jung's thought around upon itself in an effort to advance it via immanent critique. In the essay of his I am drawing upon here, it is, of course, Jung's interpretation of Christianity that is subjected to this treatment. Turning this around upon itself, Giegerich demonstrates, in the course of a thoroughgoing reflexive analysis, how on nearly every point it falls below the *niveau* of the psychological principles and interpretative standards that Jung had himself introduced into psychology and carefully applied when it was a question of other topics.

Weighed in the Scales …

It will not be necessary to précis here all the various shortcomings and excesses that Giegerich exposes in Jung's reading of Christianity. For our purposes it is enough to simply recall several of the psychological principles and interpretative standards of Jung's which Giegerich shows him to have failed to apply when it came to Christianity.

The first of these has simply to do with a clear recognition of what psychology is *about.* In "Basic Postulates of Analytical Psychology" Jung argues for a "'psychology with soul,' that is, a psychology [*Seelenlehre*] based on the hypothesis of an autonomous mind [*Geist*]" (*CW* 8 § 661, W. G.'s modified transl.).[1] With this key statement he indicates that what might variously and interchangeably be referred to as consciousness, mindedness, or the soul is not to be taken as secondary to something else which it can be reduced to, but must be seen as a reality in its own right that posits, expresses, and reflects *itself*. Concurring with Jung on this point, Giegerich in an earlier essay has given it the form of a shibboleth: "The psychological question is not, cannot be, what and how the soul is, but how the soul is reflected in its manifestations. … [P]sychology is the study of the reflection in some mirror and not the study of what the mirror is the reflection of."[2] Practically speaking, what this means is that in our work as psychologists we must not be taken in by the myriad versions of the seduction theory which psychic phenomena suggest through their sensuous, affective, and imagistic immediacy, but must form our interpretations by seeing through to what these phenomena, precisely by appearing as they do, say about the soul. Jung taught us, for example, that the incest motif does not mean incest in the

---

[1] Cited by Giegerich in *What is "Soul"?* (New Orleans: Spring Journal Books, 2012), p. 6.

[2] Wolfgang Giegerich, "Is the Soul 'Deep'? Entering and Following the Logical Movement of Heraclitus' 'Fragment 45'," *Spring* 64, pp. 1-2. Reprinted in *CEP* VI, pp. 131-132. Compared with what I have called Giegerich's shibboleth, Jung's epistemologically-couched presentation of his psychological position with respect to God and god-images is rather lax: "An archetypal image is like the portrait of an unknown man in a gallery. His name, his biography, his existence in general are unknown, but we assume nevertheless that the picture portrays a once living subject, a man who was real. We find numberless images of God, but we cannot produce the original. There is no doubt in my mind that there is an original behind our images, but it is inaccessible. We could not even be aware of the original since its translation into psychic terms is necessary in order to make it perceptible at all" (*CW* 18 §1589). With his thinking in terms of "the original" that is "behind our images" and of "translation" Jung effectively undoes the point he is making about the reflectedness of the psyche, while showing at the same time (ironically enough, since his intention was to indicate the opposite) that not only as a man, but as a psychologist, he has a God. Tacking a few words onto another of his sentences we could put it this way: just as "…one [theologian] speaks of the paradoxical God of the Old Testament, another of the incarnate God of Love, a third of the God who has a heavenly bride" (*CW* 14 § 781), so Jung speaks of what could be called his "Not God but the God-image God."

literal sense, but indicates a symbolic reality or soul truth (*CW* 16 § 419). Likewise, in *The Visions Seminars*, he argues that his patient's dream of going to visit a doctor who lives by the sea should not to be taken as a reference to him, even though he is her doctor and lives by Lake Zürich. Stating this in the form a principle he then concludes, "We should not judge dreams from realities because in the long run that leads nowhere."[3]

But what, it may be asked, can dreams and other soul texts mean if they are to be considered apart from any real referents? An important footnote in Giegerich's essay provides a "with Jung, against Jung, beyond Jung" answer to this question. In this note he works with a passage from *Answer to Job* in which Jung states the main tenet of his interpretation of Christianity. "Job," writes Jung, "... was an ordinary human being, and therefore the wrong done to him, and through him to mankind, can according to divine justice, only be repaired by an incarnation of God in an empirical human being. This act of expiation is performed by the Paraclete; for, just as man must suffer from God, so God must suffer from man. Otherwise there can be no reconciliation between the two" (*CW* 11 § 657). Now the problem with this passage, as Giegerich makes clear in the body of his essay, is that against his own rules Jung takes the figures he is dealing with for real. Though he knows well enough in other contexts that incest does not refer to actual incest and that dreams are not to be judged from realities, he here takes Job at face value as an ordinary human being and God quite literally and trans-textually as God. But this, as Giegerich rightly insists, will not do. Psychology is not about such realities as people and God (if God is indeed a reality) and not about their external relationships. Rather, it is about the soul *per se*, consciousness as such.[4] And in keeping with this its job

---

[3] C. G. Jung, *The Visions Seminars*, Book One (Zürich: Spring Publications, 1976), p. 8.

[4] The following passage from Giegerich may help to make this clearer: "For a true psychology, only the soul, which is certainly undemonstrable, merely 'metaphorical' and for this reason a seeming nothing, can be the 'substrate' and subject of the phenomena. The human being is then their object; he or she is nothing but the place where soul shows itself, just like the world is the place where man shows himself and becomes active. We therefore must shift our standpoint away from 'the human person' to the 'soul.' (*N.B.*: I am talking of

is simply to ask, as Giegerich does with respect to the passage from Jung we have just cited, "What kind of consciousness is [it] that thinks about [such and such a topic and does so, moreover, in such and such a way]?"

Now, of course, Giegerich's actual sentence is more specific than this. For didactic purposes I removed for the moment the critical reference he makes in its latter half to the ideas he had quoted from Jung. In doing so my aim has been to produce the general form of what might be called *psychology's question*. Simply by examining what this question in its general form is driving at we can gain a keener grasp of what it means to say that psychology is about the soul. But here now, having obtained this keener grasp, let us add the redacted reference to Jung's text back in. On the heels of his having cited Jung's statement about the wrong that was done to Job by God and the expiation for this that would have to be performed by the Paraclete, Giegerich derisively inveighs:

> What kind of consciousness is it that thinks about human misfortunes and terrible suffering as a "*wrong* done to him" (by God/Fate/Life) and as obviously requiring the repairing of an injustice? Do we have a vested right to be well-treated by life and to fairness? A category mistake. Behind it all is the innocent childlike belief in and demand for an ideal world and a good and just God. (*Spring* 84, p. 66; *CEP* VI, p. 182)[5]

As criticism goes this a masterstroke. Simply by keeping the focus upon what psychology is about, Jung's failure to do so himself is exposed along with something of the mindset that led

---

the shift of *our standpoint, perspective, or of the idea in terms of which* we study, just as before, the concrete experience of individuals or peoples.)" "The Present as Dimension of the Soul: 'Actual Conflict' and Archetypal Psychology," in *The Neurosis of Psychology*, *CEP*, Vol. 1, p. 115.

[5] It is interesting to note that Edinger briefly considered the same criticism: "I know when I first read *Answer to Job* when it came out in translation in the fifties, what offended me was how seriously [Jung] took this Old Testament God-image, expecting something from Him. … I thought, 'Grow up Jung, don't you realize you mustn't expect justice? The world isn't like that.'" Faithful to Jung, however, Edinger faulted himself for expressing a "rationalist position" with this objection. Edward F. Edinger, *Transformation of the God-mage: An Elucidation of Jung's Answer to Job* (Toronto: Inner City Books, 1992), p. 24.

him astray. But this is not all. A sentence later another line from Jung is quoted: "[Modern man has] experienced things so unheard of and so staggering that the question of whether such things are in any way reconcilable with the idea of a good God has become burningly topical" (*CW* 11 § 736). And then, rounding upon this sentiment, Giegerich delivers the *coup de grâce.* Far from being burningly topical, Jung's concerns as given in these statements amount to "The kindergarten idea of a good God"!!! (*Spring* 84, p. 66-67; *CEP* VI, p. 182).[6]

As asked by Giegerich, psychology's question is simply devastating. A key part of Jung's interpretation of Christianity is shown to consist of a regressive sinking of psychology back into a wishful, low-grade version of the theological/theosophical style of thinking that preceded it. This is a shocking surprise. One would have thought that the great psychologist would have known his business—thought, that is to say, that he would have asked this question himself of his biblical sources. But having failed to do so, the question rebounds upon him instead—and this, moreover, in a manner that recalls that scene of priestly succession in the Grove of Diana at Nemi that Fraser discusses in *The Golden Bough*.[7] The *coup de grâce*, indeed!

Psychology's Self-Production via Saying Again and Seeing Through

At the end of Part One, after having shown Jung's investment in the God-image (and at times, even, in a really existing God), we asked if Jungian analysis is conceivable *in absentia dei.* Already, from our brief examination of only a footnote's worth of

---

[6] To be fair to Jung, it needs to be acknowledged that in his writings he emphasized the dark side of God. This, however, does not contradict Giegerich's point. It is the other side of the same kind of thinking in terms of our vested interests and our human lot.

[7] I here follow Peter White in alluding to Sir James Frazer's account in *The Golden Bough* of the succession of priests at Nemi. See: Peter White, "Thinking 'Murder': Following the Trail of Psychology's Uroboric Knowing of Itself in No Country for Old Men," *Jung Journal: Culture & Psyche*, vol. 5, no. 2 (Spring 2011), pp. 71-83.

Giegerich's critique of Jung's reading of Christianity, the answer becomes apparent. Of course, it is. Psychology is about the soul. And this means, among many other things, that when "God" is its topic the task is to see through to what the specific God-image or God-concept indicates with respect to consciousness, what it says about "the soul."

But just here another question arises. As correct as the above statement may be (and I think that it is correct), has it not been rattled off a bit too glibly? Yes, psychology must see through. The trouble is, though, that for what Giegerich would call a truly psychological psychology to exist at all it must time and again produce itself anew through the very act of seeing through that it is supposed then to perform.

The problem I am pointing out is the problem of external reflection, or as this might also be called, of the positivity of psychology. Steering clear of these, it is of crucial importance that psychology not be thought of as field of study existing independently over and against the phenomenon it studies, as for instance the "and" in the expression "psychology *and* religion" implies. Rather, it must produce itself—as true insight tends to—through the thoughtful process of interiorizing its subject matter, whatever that may be (a text, a dream, a life situation), into itself.[8]

Drawing upon a Hegelian vocabulary, Giegerich speaks in this connection of *absolute negative interiorization*. Absolute negative interiorization is a methodological stance that stresses the

[8] There is a crucial difference for Giegerich between interiorizing a soul-phenomenon or soul-text into itself and interiorizing it into us as a supposed anthropological constant which is to be realized during the course of the individuation process. In the former case, the adept forgets about himself and becomes, as it were, for the duration of his reflective effort a sublated moment of the phenomenon that thinks itself out through him. By means of this implicit/explicit dialectic, truth is created and opened up. The later approach of interiorizing the phenomenon into oneself takes us out of psychology into the boutique of the Beautiful Soul. See in this connection Jung's reference to "glamour" at the end of the "Life after Death" chapter of *MDR* and his later reference in the same chapter to the principle of necessary statement. While this principle appears to be synonymous with the interiorizing of phenomena into themselves, the pitch is queered because of identifications that result from not having forgotten oneself and fully gone over into the phenomenon.

intrinsic interiority or self-character of any phenomenon that of its own accord has become the locus of our interest and attention. Sublated from the outset, having self-character to begin with, such phenomena are already the soul speaking about itself, already psychology, even, but of course only implicitly. They still need to be reflected into themselves, fathomed in the complexity of their mutually constituting moments, thought through to the end in order for their knowing to become explicit. And here it could be added that with these reflections Giegerich is only taking very seriously the interpretative principle that is contained in the statement of Jung's that he quotes in his essay: "What the dream, which is not manufactured by us, says is *just so*. Say in it again as well as you can" (*Letters* 2, p. 591, to Herbert Read, 2 September 1960).

Interiorizing Christianity into Itself

We are now able to address the part of Giegerich's critique that is most pertinent to the question I have raised as to the tenure of God in analytical psychology.

In his aforementioned *Tavistock Lectures* Jung told his largely Freudian audience, "My problem is to wrestle with the big monster of the historical past, the great snake of the centuries, the burden of the human mind, the problem of Christianity" (*CW* 18 § 279). In Giegerich's view, Jung had the right instinct here. While other psychologies just start directly with what they are seduced into believing psychology to be about (introspective data, personal history, or what Jung called "the joys of the cradle or a bad upbringing" [*CW* 17 § 95]), a truly psychological psychology must first reflect itself, that is, the history of its subjectivity, the history of its consciousness, and in this venture, as Jung rightly indicates, there could hardly be a worthier prime matter than the religion whose waning has most immediately preceded the rise of modern psychology in the West, the religion of Christianity.

But what in this case does "reflecting itself" mean? Historical reflection in the ordinary sense of looking back behind psychology to its Christian pre-history is only one part of it. The more important part has to do with psychology's aforementioned self-production as an interpretive discipline via saying again and seeing through. We have learned from Giegerich that "psychology is the study of the reflection in some mirror and not the study of what the mirror is the reflection of." Clarifying this further he has advised that "since the soul cannot be approached directly, … psychological investigation has to take the form of a commentary on given 'documents of the soul'."[1] Christianity, of course, is such a document, such a mirror, as is the interpretation or commentary that psychology subsequently and self-constitutively gives it. And from this the question arises as to whether the discourse of psychology is truly up to the documents it grapples with, or bringing this back to Jung, whether his interpretation does justice to the soul that is manifest in the Christianity that his psychology was developed to succeed, push off from, dream onward.[2]

We have already mentioned several of the interpretative principles of Jung's that Giegerich has drawn upon in forming his critique. There was the insistence upon a psychology "with soul" that is at the same time about the soul, the idea of psychology's producing itself by dwelling with the phenomenon and saying it again, and the cautionary remark about not explaining dreams (and other psychic phenomena) from realities. Two other statements of Jung's that Giegerich refers to throughout his work should be drawn into our discussion. The first of these has to do with what Giegerich, with the sealed retort of alchemy in mind,

---

[1] Giegerich, "Is the Soul 'Deep'?," *Spring* 64, pp. 1-2. Also, *CEP*, VI, p. 132.

[2] "Psychology, in Jung's view … *requires* otherness, difference—though not an utterly external other, something totally irrelevant, but its own internal other. Psychology must reflect itself in and base itself on a true (even if ultimately internal) other." Though Giegerich here is referring to Jung's work on alchemy it applies as well to his treatment of Christianity. As for what Giegerich means by "reflect itself and base itself on [its] true … other," this comes across in the following question he poses: "… [D]oes psychological theory do justice to the spirit of its own internal other? Did what it discovered in the latter really come home to and permeate the constitution of the former? … Is this other, [here Christianity], conceived, comprehended, and described by this theory in such a way that the "[Christian impulse]" (the inner motif power of [Christianity]) can really find fulfillment?" Wolfgang Giegerich, "Closure and Setting Free, or: The Bottled Spirit of Alchemy and Psychology," *Spring 74*, pp. 32-33. Also, *CEP*, V, p. 372.

has called systematic closure: "Above all don't let anything from outside, that does not belong, get into it, for the fantasy-image has 'everything it needs' within itself" (*CW* 14 § 749, Giegerich's transl.).[3] The second has to do with what Giegerich conceives of as the tautological self-referentiality of soul texts: "In myths and fairy tales, as in dreams, the soul speaks about itself, and the archetypes reveal themselves in their natural interplay, as 'formation, transformation / eternal Mind's eternal recreation'" (*GW* 9/1 § 400, Giegerich's transl.; cf., *CW* 9, i § 400).[4] Taken together (and they do mutually define and complement each other) these interpretative principles, gleaned from Jung's writings, are like the bands with which Odysseus had himself bound to the mast of his ship so that he could listen to the singing of the Sirens without becoming entranced by them or bewitched. Such bands, of course, are essential in any kind interpretative work, if the interpreter is not to be waylaid for too long, by some Circe or Calypso, through overvaluing one or another moment of the phenomenon that he or she holds particularly dear.

But the question arises: What happens to these constituting constraints of a truly psychological attitude when it comes to interpreting the Christian "dream" text? Again, we are surprised to be shown by Giegerich the extent to which Jung broke with key features of his own methodology. Though Jung well knew that Christianity and its history reflect the history of consciousness, writing from his emotions he treats it at the same time as if it were one of Rorschach's projective inkblots and weighs in, so to speak, with his own demand for personal meaning. The result of this, not surprisingly, is that the effort miscarries. Jung finds *his* "myth," but at the expense of the professional, "state of the art" level of psychology proper.

---

3 For a discussion of the application of systematic closure and of this principle quoted from Jung see Giegerich's essay, "Closure and Setting Free," *Spring* 74, p. 57. The same quote from Jung is discussed by Giegerich under the heading "The presupposition of the 'self-sufficiency' of myths and fantasy images" in *The Soul's Logical Life* (Frankfurt am Main, Peter Lang GmbH, 1998), p. 126.

4 For Giegerich's discussion of this passage from Jung see *The Soul's Logical Life*, p. 123. For his discussion of "The 'tautological' presupposition of myth interpretation" see pp. 119-122.

The Opus Parvum/Opus Magnum Distinction

The problem I am pointing out has to do with a blurring of the distinction between what Giegerich has called the "little work" of an individual person's individuation process and the "great work" of mankind's individuation. In the Jungian literature there is a plethora of studies in which symbols and myths from diverse traditions have been wrenched from their historical, cultural, and communal contexts and drawn into the service of illustrating archetypal dimensions of the individual development and healing of contemporary men and women. Updating Jung's dictum that "the *tertium comparationis* of all … symbol[ism] is the libido" (*CW* 5 § 329), the impression comes across that "one's personal journey," as this has come to be called, is what the myths and symbols were about in the first place.

All this, of course, began with Jung and the inspiring account he gave of the life-enhancing importance of the individual's developing a position for himself with respect to the topics that from time immemorial have been of importance to the soul. Consider, for example, the paragraphs in *Memories* that preface the setting out of his views on a topic which has traditionally gone hand in hand with belief in God, life after death. Concerned about the injury that critical rationalism has dealt the full phenomenon of human life, Jung makes a compelling case for our imaginative re-engagement with this erstwhile theme, for this as he sees it is "a healing and valid activity … [that] … gives existence a glamour which we would not like to do without."

> … A man should be able to say he has done his best to form a conception of life after death, or to create some image of it—even if he must confess his failure. Not to have done so is a vital loss. For the question that is posed to him is the age-old heritage of humanity: an archetype, rich in secret life, which seeks to add itself to our own individual life in order to make it whole. (*MDR*, p. 302)

Had Jung just left it at this, we could perhaps let his views stand uncontradicted. For it is probably true that for many people life is more personally fulfilling if a sense of its mysteries is kept alive by their imaginatively participating in them. And if, as Jung also said, our speculations concerning a life after death are only a matter of one's telling a good ghost story by the fire as one smokes a pipe, well what is the harm in that?

But Jung goes much further than this. By the end of the chapter he advises that the most rigorous of his interpretative principles, such as those ones we discussed above as being constitutive of a true psychology, should be drawn upon in this effort:

> … [I]t is all-important for a disciplined imagination to build up images of intangibles by logical principles and on the basis of empirical data, that is, on the evidence of dreams. The method employed is what I have called "the method of the necessary statement." It represents the principle of *amplification* in the interpretation of dreams …. (*MDR*, p. 310)

The problem here, as I have already indicated, is not so much that the persons Jung has in mind will not benefit from such an approach. Quite possibly they will (on an ego-security, if not ego-integrity level). The concern, rather, is about what happens to psychology (i.e., to the methodological stance of a true psychology) when the finger that applied this ointment is put back into the bottle.

We have already heard from Jung that "[i]n myths and fairy tales, as in dreams, the soul speaks about itself …." With this remark, Jung distinguishes the soul in its greater sense as consciousness *per se* or mindedness as such from the usual, personalistic sense of soul that derives from ego-determined wishes with respect to how we would like the soul to be during the various phases of the lifecycle from cradle to grave. This is a crucial distinction. Referred to by Giegerich as "the psychological difference," it is the difference between a psychology that is of the soul and about the soul and a psychology that is of and about persons, or again, between the psychic phenomena which animate a person or a people and the *truth* of those phenomena. As Giegerich has pointed out, when Jung was up to his soul-psychology/ego-psychology distinction he wrote in a manner that unfolded the psychology of the soulful phenomenon itself, be it the Trinity, the transformation symbolism of the Mass, the mythic features of U.F.O. accounts, or a schizophrenic's vision of a solar phallus.[1] Without reference to the interior of people, he worked out the logical life of those symbols that marked the horizon of the human. Just as often, however, he let the difference collapse, as when, for example, in the course of justifying his speculations concerning life after death he appealed to the fact that "for most people it means a great deal to assume that their lives will have an indefinite continuity beyond their present existence. They live more sensibly, feel better, and are more at peace" (*MDR*, p. 300).[2]

Here, it is important to realize, the consoling therapist in Jung got the better of the psychologist in him, so much so, in fact, that he even allowed his psychological method to be drawn into the service of providing comforting illusions! And this by no means is the only example of his working in such a pandering-to-the-ego manner. As Giegerich has reminded us in an earlier essay,[3] there is also Jung's story about the woman he met on his travels whose life he characterized as "... grotesquely banal, utterly poor, meaningless, with no point in it all." Put in mind by her plight of the fulfilled dignity of the Pueblo Indians he had visited in New Mexico who believed that through their ritual they helped the Sun, their father, across the sky, Jung proposed a dose of the same medicine for her:

> If she is killed today, nothing has happened, nothing has vanished—because she was nothing! But if she could say, "I am

[1] An example of Jung analyzing, not what people want in the way of life after death, but what the concept says about the soul can be found in his "Psychological Commentary on 'The Tibetan Book of the Dead'": "It is highly sensible of the *Bardo Thödol* to make clear to the dead man the primacy of the psyche, for that is the one thing which life does not make clear to us. We are so hemmed in by things which jostle and oppress that we never get a chance, in the midst of these 'given' things, to wonder by whom they are 'given.' It is from this world of 'given' things that the dead man liberates himself; and the purpose of the instruction is to help him towards this liberation" (*CW* 11 § 841).

[2] Paul Kugler has drawn attention to Jung's tendency to interpret images of the dead on the objective level, noting that this was in contravention to his own interpretive guidelines. See his "The Legacy of the Dead" in *Raids on the Unthinkable: Freudian and Jungian Psychoanalysis* (New Orleans: Spring Journal Books, 2005), pp. 120-124.

[3] Giegerich, "The End of Meaning and the Birth of Man," pp. 29-30.

> the daughter of the Moon. Every night I must help the Moon, my Mother, over the horizon"—ah, that is something else! Then she lives, then her life makes sense, and makes sense in all continuity, and for the whole of humanity. That gives peace, when people feel that they are living the symbolic life, that they are actors in the divine drama. That gives the only meaning to human life; everything else is banal and you can dismiss it. A career, producing of children, are all *maya* compared with that one thing, that your life is meaningful. (*CW* 18 § 630)

Reading this passage one can only admire the prescience of Freud's warning to Jung, during the course of their very first meeting in 1907, about the danger of releasing, in the name of analysis, a "black tide of mud … of occultism" (*MDR*, p. 150). For that is what this Daughter of the Moon therapy amounts to, a tide of consoling illusions which no doubt are quite comforting to the Beautiful Soul as it tightens up against that animus moment of the syzygy which, unrecognized as such by Jung, was vilified by him as the soul-less rationalism of the contemporary critical mind and modern world.

But the point I want to make has to do with the deleterious effect that this pandering to the ego and vilifying of the critical mind had upon Jung's principles of interpretation even after his consulting room was closed for the day and he was working over biblical texts in his study. In his preface to *Answer to Job* Jung makes a virtue of the fact that he was unable to write the book "in a coolly objective manner," but allowed his "emotional subjectivity to speak" (*CW* 11 § 559). Underscoring this point, he characterizes himself as having written out of a sense of provocation. Outraged by Yahweh's immoral treatment of Job, he drew inspiration from his own "equally ill-considered outburst of affect" and "smouldering resentment," "… express[ing] his affect fearlessly and ruthlessly … and … answer[ing] injustice with injustice" (*CW* 11 § 561). Quite rightly Giegerich asks, "Why does [Jung] write a book about a topic when he is still personally gripped by its 'numinosity'? Why did he not see it as his obligation as a psychologist to work off (to have long ago worked off for himself) this 'numinous' affect and overcome his feeling 'wounded' by it?" (*CEP*, Vol. IV, p. 195, note 12)

Later in his Job book Jung again judges and rewrites the biblical text in terms of affects, desires, and subjective reactions as, for instance, when he takes the text-external "deep longing in the masses for an intercessor and mediatrix who would at last take her place alongside the Holy Trinity and be received as the 'Queen of Heaven and Bride at the heavenly court'" (*CW* 11 § 748) as an authenticating touchstone of his revisionist reading of Christianity. Just like the woman he had met on his travels whose life, supposedly, would have been worthwhile if she could have said "I am the daughter of the Moon," so, thanks to the papal declaration of 1950, can the Catholic faithful find meaning in the Dogma of the Assumption of Mary and *Da Vinci Code* Jungians in the Sophia Jung imports from Proverbs and Ecclesiastes into his account of the Job story.[4]

Again, it is apparent from this that the therapist in Jung got the better of the depth psychologist in him. Rather than giving his heart and mind fully over to the task of dispassionately fathoming what the text's being as it is says about the soul, he imposes a subjectively conditioned politically correct make-over upon it that is designed to met people's needs, e.g., for a good God, a metaphysical representation of the feminine, the resacralization of the secular, and whatnot. It is the exact opposite of Giegerich's insistence, in the spirit of alchemy, that as psychologists "our Christianity is not the people's Christianity." Jung's intent, by contrast, was to provide a psychology for the people. Even though he "strictly distinguished" between "the psychology of the religious person" and "the psychology of religion proper, i.e., of religious contents" and claimed that it was "chiefly [his] experiences in the latter field which [had] given [him] the courage to enter into the discussion of the religious question …" (*CW* 11 § 751-752), he nevertheless got his wires crossed, such that his soul psychology was more personalistic than he realized. For, indeed, on his analysis, religion belonged not to the *intelligible* soul as its (now antiquated) mode of speaking about itself, but to people as their immediately felt, meaning-providing, self-validating experience.

---

[4] For a related critique of this topic see W. Giegerich, "The 'Patriarchal Neglect of the Feminine Principle': A Psychological Fallacy in Jungian Theory." *Harvest: Journal for Jungian Studies*, vol. 45, no. 1 (1999), pp. 7-30. Also, *CEP*, Vol. VI, pp. 47-84.

The Beautiful Soul and Its Too-Terrible-to-Be-True Other

Passing mention was made above of the Beautiful Soul. The term itself comes from Hegel (amongst others) who used it to describe a determination of consciousness, typical of the Romantics but by no means exclusive to them, wherein the subject self-identically clings to innocence and purity by tightening up against the world or something bad within it that has been constituted as such out of all that offends its sense of soul. Closer to our own time, and with specific reference to Jung, this same problematic has been reformulated by Philip Rieff as what he calls "the triumph of the therapeutic."[1] In contrast to Freud, who had emphasized the disenchanting of neurosis via the analytic attitude, Jung is shown by Rieff to have sought a cure for his patients by means of "a meta-religion aiming at something beyond the criteria of true and false, or even good and evil …" and whose "… ideal character type … is neither mystic nor ascetic, but therapeutic—a person assessing even his own myth in terms of how much it contributes to his sense of personal well-being."[2]

In support of Rieff's contention any number of passages could be cited. The one that comes most immediately to my mind (next to the life after death and daughter of the Moon material discussed above) is from Jung's essay, "Psychology and Religion":

> Religious experience is absolute; it cannot be disputed. You can only say that you have never had such an experience, whereupon your opponent will reply: "Sorry, I have." And there your discussion will come to an end. No matter what the world thinks about religious experience, the one who has it possesses a great treasure, a thing that has become for him a source of life, meaning, and beauty, and that has given a new splendour to the world and to mankind. He has *pistis* and peace. Where is the criterion by which you could say that such a life is not legitimate, that such an experience is not valid, and that such

---

[1] Philip Rieff, *The Triumph of the Therapeutic: Uses of Faith after Freud* (New York, Harper & Row, 1966).

[2] *Ibid*, pp. 113-114.

> *pistis* is mere illusion? Is there, as a matter of fact, any better truth about the ultimate things than the one that helps you to live? (*CW* 11 § 167)

The first sentences of this passage declare religious experience to be intrinsically authoritative, immediately self-validating and as such immune from criticism, unanswerable. In the conversation described by Jung, discussion is stopped short when the one party smugly asserts that he has had a religious experience—and that that's all there is to it. Evidently, for Jung, there is no need for any rational accounting with respect to a religious experience. No need for any "trying of the spirits" to see if the experience is true.[3] With the middle sentences we are taken a little farther down the same path. Religious experience is set up as something to be treasured over and against what the world of others thinks. We may be reminded in this connection of Jung's insistence in *The Undiscovered Self* upon the individual's need of "the evidence of inner, transcendental experience which alone can protect him from the otherwise inevitable submersion in the [social, collective] mass." According to this view, "… an extramundane principle capable of relativizing the overpowering influence of external factors" is needed to safeguard one's "spiritual and moral autonomy," for "the individual who is not anchored in God can offer no resistance on his own resources to the physical and moral blandishments of the world" (*CW* 10 § 511). God, as referred to in these lines, is not the immanent depth of one's total situation, not the inwardness and universality of the matter at hand, but one's own affects or affect images produced as wholly other to oneself and trumped up into a sort of Archimedean position-like anthropological constant and eternal verity.[4] As for the last sentences of the cited passage, with these

[3] 1 John 4:1. Cf. Giegerich's reference to "… 'trying the spirits,' whether they are in accordance with the developed constitution of psychology or not." *The Neurosis of Psychology*, *CEP*, Vol. 1, p. 7.

[4] With reference to my stating that "one's own affects or affect images … [are] *produced as* wholly other to oneself," the following passage from Jung is quite telling: "… [A]ll modern people feel alone in the world of the psyche because they assume that there is nothing there that they have not made up. … *But through a certain training* … something suddenly happens which one has not

the picture of the Beautiful Soul as it pertains to Jung's psychology is fully drawn. Clutching onto some affective experience as to a numinous talisman, the religiously-cathected analysand tinkers with the checks and balances of his personal well-being, there being, as Jung avers, "no better truth … than the one that helps you to live."[5]

But is it really so that there is no better truth than this? Jung quoted with approval the adage that "the good is always the enemy of the better" (*CW* 17 § 320). Could this not be applied to Jung's religio-therapeutic pragmatism? Is what it offers not at best a good? And as this good, is it not the enemy of that (sometimes terrible) better, truth itself?

A passage of Nietzsche's is helpful here in releasing Jung's psychology from the mandalated ethos of personal well-being in which it has come to be cocooned:

> How many people still make the inference: "one could not stand life if there were not God!" (or as they say in the circles of the Idealists: "one could not stand life if it lacked the ethical significance of its ground!")—consequently there *must* be a God (or an ethical significance of existence)! … What presumption to decree that all that is necessary for my preservation must also really *be there*! As if my preservation were anything necessary![6]

There could hardly be a more chastening critique than this. Once again the philosopher with a hammer percusses a treasured

---

created, something objective, and then one is no longer alone. That is the object of [certain] initiations, *to train people to experience something which is not their intention*, something strange, something objective with which they cannot identify… This experience of the objective fact is all-important, because it denotes the presence of something which is not I, yet is still psychical. Such an experience can reach a climax where it becomes an experience of God." *The Visions Seminars*, Book One (Zürich: Spring Publications, 1976), p. 73, italics mine.

[5] As for Jung's bluster-filled challenge— "Where is the criterion by which you could say that such a life is not legitimate, that such an experience is not valid, and that such *pistis* is mere illusion?"—it can readily be argued that the paragraph from which this is taken is itself the criterion by which Jung judged the life of the woman he met on his travels to be "… grotesquely banal, utterly poor, meaningless, with no point in it all."

[6] Cited by Walter Kaufmann in *Nietzsche: Philosopher, Psychologist, Antichrist*, 3rd ed. (New York: Vintage Books, 1968), p. 356.

human value and shows it to be hollow. But there is more to these lines of Nietzsche's than even he saw. This becomes evident when we read them with Giegerich's insights concerning the animus as negation and as the soul's own other in mind. In *Dialectics & Analytical Psychology* and, again, in *Soul-Violence*, Giegerich makes the crucial point that animus figures such as Hades and Bluebeard are not external others with respect to the anima figures they threaten, but rather, their very own internal syzygial counterparts.[7] Read in this light the sentiment at the beginning of Nietzsche's text — "one could not stand life if there were not God … consequently there *must* be a God"—is the innocent *anima alba* moment of the syzygy while the later remark about the presumption of decreeing that what is necessary for my preservation must also really be there is the negating (killing, raping, disillusioning) animus moment. And from this it follows that what I am calling the animus-aspect of Nietzsche's text (and we can expand this to include his announcement of the death of God!) is not some kind of spoiling, extraneous incursion of abstract atheism, but the moment of immanent critique wherein the innocent initial position loses its innocence through being as fully and seriously applied as was, if I may put it this way, the feline curiosity that killed the proverbial cat. Prior to this, it must be said, there was no animus. The animus, after all, is not a being or thing. It has no separate existence, but only exists as the wounding realization that what seemed to be the case no longer is so, if ever it was.[8] Bringing this point back to our passage from Nietzsche, there were in earlier times whole ages in which such a critical reflection would have been just as preposterous as he rightly makes our clinging to God seem today. Why? Because, like Thor appearing whenever there was a giant to be grappled with or an ordeal to be surpassed, the Gods were there! Nietzsche's text, by contrast, speaks from a time and into a time in which all this has changed.

---

[7] Wolfgang Giegerich, David L. Miller, Greg Mogenson, *Dialectics & Analytical Psychology: The El Capitan Canyon Seminar* (New Orleans: Spring Journal Books, 2005), pp. 108-112. Wolfgang Giegerich, "The Animus as Negation and as the Soul's Own Other," in *CEP*, Vol. III, pp. 111-167.

[8] Giegerich, "The Animus as Negation," *CEP*, Vol. III, pp. 112-113, 144-145, 147.

And what of this change? A passage from an essay of Giegerich's titled "Rupture, Or: Psychology and Religion" is most pertinent in this connection. Writing with reference to the soul's having gone through fundamental changes as a function of time,[9] Giegerich speaks of a "rupture [having] taken place." This, he explains (with especially the 18th and 19th centuries in mind), "… consist[s] in the fact that the world to which the known religions were answers has, as it were, *moved out from under them*," such that "… we are now confronted with a logically entirely new world, to which religion no longer corresponds."[10] Continuing some pages later he adds:

> I would … not ask what we can expect from religion and what concrete measures need to be taken to realize our expectations. I would not [suggest we] think about how to rescue our various religious traditions and bring them over into the changed world of today. For any such attempt would in my eyes only amount to an attempt to rescue the logical status or level of consciousness that we are subjectively living in and comfortably accustomed to and to freeze us psychologically in the past, while objectively we have for long been living in a reality characterized by a new logical status. The rupture in the objective world out there necessitates a corresponding rupture in us, and in us not as persons, but as the logic or psychology as which we live. It is not enough to try to adapt our religions to our new situation, it is not them that have to be adjusted. It is us. And this is why I think the answer to the problem of religion in our contemporary world is "psychology"—not psychology as a particular science, as this or that school of thought, but psychology as a move to be made, the move of turning the question of religion back onto ourselves, onto that which is closest to us: our status of consciousness; in other words, psychology as the realization of the unavoidable necessity of the death to be died by our frame of mind.[11]

---

[9] Time, in this context, needs to be understood, not as an external factor, but as the animus moment of the soul's syzygy. Critical of what he calls "anima-only" psychology, Giegerich has re-acquainted Jungian and archetypal psychology with the animus of history.

[10] Wolfgang Giegerich, "Rupture, or: Psychology and Religion" in *CEP*, Vol. I, p. 227, italics mine.

[11] *Ibid.* pp. 229-230.

The Rupture in the Soul

With his reference to "… a rupture [having] taken place … [wherein] … the world to which the known religions were answers has … *moved out from under them*," Giegerich soberly describes the situation Nietzsche spoke of when he issued his spectacular announcement regarding the death of God. Jung, of course, for his part also knew about this rupture. He knew, that is to say, that "we are living in what the Greeks called the καιρος—the right moment—for a 'metamorphosis of the gods,' of the fundamental principles and symbols" (*CW* 10 § 585). In a letter to Fr. White he even went so far as to declare that "we are actually living in the time of the splitting of the world and the invalidation of Christ" (*Letters* 2, p. 138, 24 November, 1953). But haunted by the diagnosis he had affixed to Nietzsche as its foremost casualty, he also resisted this development, as when, for example, a few sentences later in the same letter he reassures his Dominican friend that "Christ is still the valid symbol. Only God can 'invalidate' himself through the Paraclete." And then there is that line from "The Symbolic Life" that we mentioned earlier about his wanting "a situation in which that thing [that had previously been mediated by Christian symbolism] becomes true once more … [in] a new form" (*CW* 18 § 632). Reflecting upon these references we can again appreciate the aptness of Giegerich's characterization of Jung's position as "God Must Not Die!"

But why, it may be asked, did Jung insist that what had formerly been the form of truth—God and the religions—be true once more in the (not really so) "new form" of revisionist theosophizing? Why, to say it with that line from Hölderlin that David Miller has reminded us of,[1] could he not allow God's absence to help us into the opaque depths of our new situation, so that we could meet its true character with open and active minds?

The answer to this question is a least twofold. On one hand, Jung upheld the validity of the Christ symbol, even at a time that

[1] "… [U]ntil God's absence helps!" This line from Hölderlin is adapted as the title to Miller's contribution to the discussion of Giegerich's article. *Spring* 84, pp. 73-90.

he recognized to objectively involve its invalidation, due to his concerns about the unleashing of primitive, atavistic impulses:

> At a time when a large part of mankind is beginning to discard Christianity, it may be worth our while to try to understand why it was accepted in the first place. It was accepted as a means of escape from the brutality and unconsciousness of the ancient world. As soon as we discard it, the old brutality returns in force, as has been made overwhelmingly clear by contemporary events. ... It is the same with individuals who lay aside one form of adaptation and have no new form to turn to: they infallibly regress along the old path and then find themselves at a great disadvantage, because the world around them has changed considerably in the meantime. (*CW* 5 § 341)

As for Jung's other reason for upholding the form of God and the validity of the Christ symbol (even at a time when the soul, in its animus moment, was turning against these forms of itself), this I submit is clearly expressed in a section of *Aion* that anticipates the interpretation that he later put forward in *Answer to Job*. Deeply concerned about "the splitting of our world" (by which he meant the divide between the conventional Christian God-image and the "sinister-realities" of the modern world that are not covered by that image and that lead to materialism, atheism and other substitutes of the like), Jung issued an uncanny warning, sounded an ominous alarm:

> ... *[T]he destruction of the God-image is followed by the annulment of the human personality.* (*CW* 9, ii § 170; Jung's italics)

No wonder Jung equivocated with regard to the invalidation of Christ that he himself had announced. No wonder he continued to insist upon the soul's having the form of God even after the death of God had been symbolically figured in the Christian "dream" text, and upon his teaching that the demise of this form led straight away to inflation, brutality, or to an ism of some sort. Nietzsche may have mocked, as he did in the passage we quoted, but it truly would be too terrible—this seems to have been Jung's view—if there were no God. And to prove this point Jung never tired of holding up the insane Nietzsche as the prime exemplar of the annulment of the personality that follows the destruction of the God-image. This, however, was hardly credible. Nietzsche's insanity was not the result of his attacking Christianity, but of an organic disease process. Jung's use of him as "exhibit A" was, thus, just another variant of that trivial joke one sees from time to time scratched upon a desktop in a classroom or lecture hall, the one in which the statement, "'God is Dead'—Nietzsche," is contradicted by the statement, "'Nietzsche is Dead'—God." Never mind that for complex epistemological reasons Jung's Nietzsche-killing deity had to be an encapsulated in reservations and caveats Not-God-but-the-God-Image-in-me God. With this strange angel the Apostle of the God-image believed he had found his "new form."

Figures of Negation

"The Rupture in the Soul," "The Split in the World," "The Invalidation of Christ," and "The Death of God": as various as these terms and topics may seem, they are at the same time synonymous with one another as figures of negation. In a discussion of this concept, so key to his own contribution to psychology, Giegerich has pointed out that while the imagining mind apperceives negation as some terrible incursion and violent action inflicted from the outside, actually and in truth it is merely the mind-internal, and yet world-embracing, recognition that the matter of interest, whatever that may be, "has all along *not* been what it had seemed …."[1]

With this in mind let us look again at the anxiety-image that underpins Jung's interpretation of Christianity. Arising from feelings that would have taken the likes of an Edvard Munch to paint, the main thrust of Jung's psychology project has had to do with averting a catastrophe both psychic and spiritual, the aforementioned annulment of the human personality, which he pictured as being consequent upon the destruction of the God-image. Reflecting upon this ominous prospect as upon the foil of his theory-making, we may be struck by the similarity of its

[1] Wolfgang Giegerich, "'The Unassimilable Remnant'—what is at Stake? A dispute with Stanton Marlan" in S. Marlan, ed., *Archetypal Psychologies: Reflections in Honor or James Hillman* (New Orleans: Spring Journal Books, 2008), p. 219.

fantasy-structure to that of persecutory pursuit-type dreams. Menaced by new truth, the figure of the dreamer in such dreams "conservatively adheres to the earlier attitude" (*CW* 4 § 350, modified), even as it frantically escapes to safety.[2] In Jung's case, the truth by which he was menaced was that of an increasingly godless present. Rather than exposing himself to this stark mystery and allowing its negating action to redefine what soul means at our present historical locus, he clung to the familiar, to the old religious definition of soul, with the aim of carrying this forward into our times. Ensconced in the safety of this effort (for what is the ire of a few theological critics compared to the godless void he feared?), the issue for him was all about keeping the tradition vital and the personality intact. And it was to this end that he advised his fellow "advocates of Christianity" not to "squander their energies in the mere preservation of what has come down to them," but to join him in the work of "building on to their house and making it roomier. [For] stagnation in these matters threatens in the long run with a lethal end" (*CW* 9, ii § 170).

But the lethal end, if one wants to call it that, had already come. Indeed, it had been operative from the outset. As the Bible puts it, on a cross in Jerusalem, God had died. For the psychologist, however, this was an *image-internal* destruction of the God-image, its internal corruption and self-sublation. Its own doing, as Giegerich would say. Far from being the result of any stagnation, it was in itself fecund, as the vast cultural achievements that Christianity unfolded from this thought amply attest.

"Our passage," writes Giegerich (with Phil. 2:5-8 in mind), "tells of one powerful dynamic, one vigorous movement of going under":

> The incarnation is not only about Christ's being *born* as man ("Christmas") in the sense of a one-time event, as it appears to the merely imagining mind. It is continued beyond his birth and goes through his life on earth as a whole right into his death. The incarnation is a complete going under and is only fulfilled with his crucifixion. And not even with this crucifixion as such alone, but only with its culminating in his absolute loss of God ("My God, my God, why hast thou forsaken me?"), which is

---

[2] Wolfgang Giegerich, *Working with Dreams: Initiation into the Soul's Speaking about Itself* (Abingdon, New York: Routledge, 2020), pp. 141-149.

> not mentioned in our passage. Only with this experience or insight had the *kenôsis* become absolute. Only then was the last trace of divinity truly emptied out. As long as there was trust in God Father and the faith or hope that he, Jesus Christ, was God's son, his child, did he indirectly still possess his divinity, even if he did not possess it immediately in himself (who had in fact already become nothing but human), but in his other, God, and in his faith in Him. The complete *kenôsis* includes the death of God, the loss of "having" a God altogether. Without the loss of God it would only be a partial or token "emptying." And only if he has lost his God has he really, unreservedly, become human, nothing but human, and emptied his cup fully. (*CEP* VI, p. 176)

Against Jung's restorative/revisionist reading of Christianity, which by his own lights was an attempt to make the Christian house roomier, Giegerich does not offer another interpretation, one of his own. Rather, with the likes of Hegel, Altizer, Jüngel, Žižek, Cupitt, and St. Paul before any of these, he "sticks to the image"—saves the phenomenon—of God's fully becoming man even as he dies as one.

The issue here, as I have been stressing throughout, is a methodological one. When St. Paul wrote to the Philippians of Christ's incarnation as his humbling himself, he did so for methodological reasons, that is, to teach the Christian ethic. The idea was that the Christian individual was to overcome his self-importance and petty jealousies, to empty himself of these even as Christ did on an even larger scale when he divested himself of his divinity and died on the cross as a man. And here it may be noted that far from annulling the human personality, the negation or destruction of the God-image that was figured in this text imparted to it its universality within the soul's new logic or successor notion, i.e., as the life "in Christ."

Now it is important to notice, further to this, that what Giegerich pointed out in his "Rupture: Or Psychology of Religion" essay with regard to our contemporary situation as a post-Enlightenment secular society was also true at that earlier rupture point at which the Christian aeon began. Then, too, a rupture in the objective world out there had necessitated a corresponding rupture in the people. "And Jesus cried out again with a loud voice and yielded up his spirit. And behold, the curtain of the temple was torn in two, from top to bottom. And the earth shook, and the rocks were split" (Matt. 27:50-51, ESV). But as Giegerich has stressed, such ruptures are not to be thought of as running through the people as persons (they are not their *fault*!); rather, they have to do with the objective character of the times, with the truth of the situation that was then prevailing. Or putting this distinction another way, we could say with Giegerich that it is not the psychology that the people *have* that is ruptured in the sense of some sort of intrapsychic dissociation; rather, rupture here refers to the liminal character of the logic or psychology which a person or a people *exists as*, or again, to be more specific, to the status of a reflecting consciousness which, being reflective, has broken with and emancipated itself from the immediacy of sense certainty, *participation mystique*, and what had formerly been its naïve relation to what it had been able to regard and propitiate as external to itself.

With these reflections we come to the crux of Giegerich's dispute with Jung. Frightened, as we have said, by what he variously called "the split in the world," "the invalidation of Christ," and "the annulment of the human personality," Jung propped up the form of God by divinizing human development and shoving it into that place where the reality of the world had been before it had "moved out from under" the religions which had become obsolete and redundant. I refer here, on one hand, to the erstwhile psychologist's identification of the Christian idea of incarnation with the personal individuation process (e.g., "'incarnation' … on the human level appears as 'individuation'" *CW* 11 § 233) and, on the other, to his experiences in active imagination of self-deification and his interpretation of these as imparting "immortal value to the individual."[3] In Jung's view, the personal relationship to the soul as God was simply indispensable. And even if now in the modern situation God needed the (graven!) images of the human individuation process to shore him up, he still remained a mighty enough reality to leave Jung wondering "… why the human frame is not shattered by the

---

[3] Jung, *Analytical Psychology: Notes of the Seminar Given in 1925*, pp. 96-97.

incarnation … [since] man with all his external characteristics seems little suited to representing a god" (*MDR*, p. 337, transl. modif.). So another fear cropped up. The remedy Jung had proposed for what he saw as the problem of the annulment of the personality—individuation—has an equally terrible side effect, the shattering of the human frame! And here, in this contradiction, we see the faultiness of the imaginal mode of thought, its tendency to literalize negation and apperceive it as external, rather than letting itself be emptied ("annulled," "shattered") and go under into the fluidity of a thinking consciousness with the realization that the content of its reflection has "… all along *not* been what it had seemed ...."[4]

It could have been different. There could have been another way. Instead of belatedly attempting to stave off the rupture in the soul by collapsing the psychological difference and inserting a miniaturized version of it into the inner of the individual person (as Jung did with his emphasis upon individuation, personal growth, and an ego-transcending Self that was nevertheless in us), the divine process of incarnation, *kenôsis*, and death could have found its successor form in the methodological stance of a truly psychological psychology.

I say "could have" here not to be wistful (though I do consider our collective striving for a truly psychological method to be a more important endeavour than our personal "Striving for Wholeness"). My point, rather, is to highlight the fact that Giegerich's critique of Jung, both in his "God Must Not Die!" essay and in many other works, is rooted in essential impulses of Jung's concept of psychological reality which Jung himself had been unable to house in his overall theory except as menacing spectres to be in flight from.

So the question arises: How is Jungian analysis to be awakened from the persecutory-pursuit dream which it enacts in its theory? Or, to be more specific, how is it to allow such menacing spectres as "the destruction of the God-image," "the annulment of the personality," "the shattering of the human frame," and, of course, the modern plight of meaninglessness to find their place within it?

---

[4] Giegerich, "'The Unassimilable Remnant'," p. 219. Also, *CEP* IV, p. 472.

In a discussion of persecutory-pursuit-type dreams Giegerich has insightfully argued that if what the dream has imaginatively presented as separate, externally-related dream-figures are grasped in their simultaneity as the refracted moments of a single, inclusive thought, the realization may dawn that what had at first been pictured and experienced as menace, on one hand, and terrified flight, on the other, is not only ultimately compatible, but has all along been, even while it perused and escaped itself, the first immediacy of the *coniunctio*. For the real *coniunctio* is not some idealized representation of unity before which the subject stands unscathed, but rather has to do with the figure of the other having really rattled one's cage, gotten under one's skin, and cut into values that one had been attempting at all costs to preserve.[5]

Jung, of course, was well aware of this dynamic, at least insofar as it figured in the lives of his patients. He knew, for example, about how menacing it could be when at the turning points of life "the greater figure, which one always was but which remained invisible, appears to the lesser personality with the force of a revelation" (*CW* 9, i § 217). The trouble, however, was with the application of his insights about this to psychological consciousness itself. When it was only a matter of a patient's neurosis or self-development, he could tough-mindedly interpret the challenge that the patient's encounter with his or her shadowy other was about, as for instance when he wrote, further to the line that we just quoted, that "he who is truly and hopelessly little will always drag the revelation of the greater down to the level of his littleness, and will never understand that the day of judgment for his littleness has dawned [while] … the man who is inwardly great will know that the long expected friend of his soul, the immortal one, has now really come, 'to lead captivity captive,' that is, to seize hold of him by whom this immortal had always been confined and held prisoner, and to make his life flow into the greater life—a moment of deadliest peril!" (*ibid.*). But after reading Giegerich's contribution to this volume we have to realize that Jung fell foul of his own insight as far as the constitution of his psychology was concerned. I refer here to those uncanny guests that his theory could not house.

[5] Giegerich, *Working with Dreams*, pp. 146-149.

In the persecutory-dream to which his theory may be likened, Jung again and again dragged the revelation of the greater, which he met in such terrifying figures as "the destruction of the God-image" and "the annulment of the human personally," down to the level of his littleness by taking flight from these into revisionist, restorative, theosophical counter-ideas such as the quaternity and the Self, Sophia and the Daughter of the Moon. Though, of course, this flight also indicates that he had to some extent also been reached by what he fled, he was nevertheless able to shield his overall conception of the soul from this by assigning the *coniunctio* to the individual as *his* task.[6]

Kenôsis as Method

In league with Giegerich, I have just characterized psychology's having foisted *its* individuation tasks off upon the individual as an example of psychology's "drag[ging] the revelation of the greater down to the level of [its] littleness, and … [not] understand[ing[that the day of judgement for [its] littleness has dawned." Bringing these reflections to a close, let us briefly discuss the alternative to this wherein psychology recognizes, in the very shadows that menace it, "the long expected friend of [*its*] soul … and make[s] [its] life flow into the greater life …."

Jung, as we know, set up a miniaturized version of the psychological difference in the inner of the individual as his vis-à-vis with the God-image in the individuation process. The alterative to this happens on the theoretical plane or notional level. Referred to by Giegerich as "the soul's logical life," the

---

[6] Commenting upon what he has called "the neurosis of psychology" Giegerich has alerted us to "[t]he innocent tendency to focus on cases and on psychological material before consciousness [which] keeps psychology unconscious about the fact that the theory (or theories, in the plural) that guide its consciousness are always in on it, from the outset." Continuing, he writes, "What should actually be the intrinsic *form of the constitution* of psychology is reduced to *empirical events* occurring in the course of the practice of psychology. The empirical persons have to carry the load that psychology as theory or logical constitution of psychology does not want to shoulder." *The Neurosis of Psychology*, *CEP*, Vol. I, p. 9.

individuation process of this, let us call it, the psychology we exist as, has to do with the self-constituting flow of psychology (in the sense of that "... most complex of psychic structures, a man's philosophy of life ..." *CW* 16 § 180) into the greatness of its concept which occurs when the psychological difference (and the negations that mediate it) is understood in its most radical sense as the difference between psychological consciousness, on one hand, and people's psychologies, on the other, or again, between the methodological stance of a truly psychological psychology and the individuation process as it occurs in people.

But how, it may be asked, is this turn to be taken wherein the negations that Jung took so literally and sought to stave off therapeutically can be understood as mediating a more radical sense of the psychological difference, and along with this, an even greater conception of psychology and the soul?

In a line that can be read as the application of Jung's seminal insight about psychology's lack of an objective, extra-psychic vantage point to this question, Giegerich avers that "... psychology begins where any phenomenon (whether physical or mental, 'real' or fantasy image) is interiorized absolute-negatively into itself, and I find myself in its internal infinity. This is what it takes; psychology cannot be had for less."[1] Underscoring this point he declares in another passage that "what at first appears as a content [or object] of consciousness is in truth the seed of what wants to become a new form of consciousness at large."[2]

Apropos of these statements, and with the help of a few more quotations from Giegerich, it is not difficult to show how the negating spectres which had so troubled Jung can be absolute negatively interiorized into themselves such that their character as the new form of consciousness and beginning point of a true psychology is disclosed. Take, for example, that terror of the soul that was propitiated by Jung as "the annulment of the human personality." When regarded as an internal other and absolute negatively interiorized into itself this menacing prospect is productive, not of the individuation process that Jung would have

---

[1] Giegerich, "Is the Soul 'Deep'?," p. 31. Also, *CEP*, Vol. IV, pp. 161-162.

[2] *Ibid.*, p. 19. Also, *CEP*, Vol IV, p. 149.

it spur on, but of an indispensable feature of a truly psychological stance: the negation of the ego. As Giegerich explains,

> [Psychological discourse] has to *be as* the negation of the ego, and the psychologist (of course only to the extent that he truly is a psychologist and speaks psychologically) has to speak as one who has long died as ego personality. The art of psychological discourse is to speak as someone already deceased.[3]

We can see from this passage that the personality is not annulled. On the contrary, having been superseded by Giegerich's insight that the psychologist must speak as someone who is already deceased, the prospect that it might be is shown to have been but the first immediacy of a *psychological consciousness* and *methodological stance* in which the ego-personality (which, as we know, is the principal subscriber of the Beautiful Soul fallacy) has no place and "the notion of soul is logically released from its attachment to the notion of the human being."[4]

There was another worry mentioned by Jung. This had to do with dissociative pathology operative on the collective level, i.e., that neurosis of our times which he referred to as "the split in our world." Open to the inner infinity of the phenomenon that this expression describes, Giegerich writes:

> … [N]eurosis is not at all the simple fact of a split. It is more complicated. The neurotic dissociation is a disunity plus its denial. … In other words, the neurotic dissociation consists in the *denial* of *itself* (of the dissociation) and, therefore, in the insistence that each of the dissociated partial truths be the whole truth. Therefore the "cure" of neurosis cannot consist in ridding us of the disunity and making us "whole" again in this sense. To assume this would not only be naïve, *the one-sided insistence on harmony and unambiguous identity is also precisely what makes for neurosis.* Not the split, but the ideal of undialectical unity is what is behind neurosis.[5]

---

[3] Giegerich, *The Soul's Logical Life*, p. 24.
[4] *Ibid.*, from the back-cover text.
[5] *Ibid.*, p. 25.

Though neurosis, disunity, dissociation, rupture and splitting are usually regarded as mere contents of consciousness, Giegerich argues that in our time they have an overarching, objective character. Indicative of that cut which consciousness inflicts upon itself through its being conscious of itself, they must even be given their dignity as the prevailing form of consciousness at large. As Giegerich explains:

> If psychology (as theory or consciousness) does not allow for division of itself, it inevitably has to project it out [such that it becomes merely the individual's task—G.M.]. No, the cure of neurosis consists in the cure of a consciousness fixated on continuity, unity, positivity, self-identity; it consists in allowing the split *to come home to* consciousness and to permeate the logical form of its constitution, in order for consciousness to become something that can give the disunity (in ourselves, in the world, in life) as well as the individual dissociated partial truths each their own legitimate place ....[6]

It only remains to bring "the destruction of the God-image" into the ambit of these reflections. Menaced by the prospect of such destruction, the cornerstone of Jung's therapeutics has had to do with revivifying the relation with the God-image by amplifying and interpreting all manner of images as God-images. Unable to see the destruction of this image, which he accurately described, as the soul's own doing and to let the rupture that this expressed come home to consciousness, he even went so far as to declare, as he put it in his *Red Book*, that "*God is an image, and those who worship him must worship him in the image of the supreme meaning.*"[7] But this line was written at a time when the death of God, which had already occurred at the inception of Christianity, had been raised to the power of two by Nietzsche among others such that consciousness at large had already long been emancipated from having to have the form of God. Jung, however, could not accept the empty sepulchre that his times had become. And so, countering this, he resurrected and restored a plethora of decorative and therapeutic Gods.

---

[6] *Ibid.*

[7] Jung, *The Red Book: Liber Novus*, p. 229.

The task of a true psychology would have been precisely the opposite of this. It would have been soulfully to *think* "the destruction of the God-image" without succumbing to either Jung's theosophizing or Nietzsche's nihilism, which is also to say, to allow the kenôtic movement of the death of God idea to permeate consciousness such that the soul, having released itself from the divine vestment that had been befitting for it in earlier times, can achieve a new definition of itself *extra ecclesiam, post mortem Dei.*

So, what are we left with? Having let so much of the positivity of Jung's psychology go under, what is it that remains? A new ability to be with that nothing that sees everything? A consciousness that can *think* rupture, rather than merely suturing it closed again with a syncretistic hodgepodge of images, myths, and meanings?

Writing with reference to an insight of Augustine's, Jung acknowledged the saint to have "apprehended a great truth, namely that every spiritual truth gradually turns into something material, becoming no more than a tool in the hand of man." Drawing the conclusion from this, he continues: "In consequence, man can hardly avoid seeing himself as a knower, yes even as a creator, with boundless possibilities at his command" (*CW* 13 § 302). Taking this insight further than the Jung who feared annulment would have been able to credit,[8] could it also be the case that that greatest of all spiritual truths, God, has become something material (or methodological), "a tool in the hand of man"?

A passage from Giegerich's "Rupture, or: Psychology and Religion" essay well conveys the substance of this soul-*making* tool. Constituted by the very emptiness of the hands that hold it, it is the notionally determined and negatively intensive methodological stance or analytic attitude of a truly psychological psychology. As Giegerich puts it:

---

[8] At the end of the same paragraph from which this line is taken, Jung vilifies the light of man's intellect for bringing about a *Götterdämmerung*.

We have to learn to *suffer* our hands to be empty, in the fullest sense of the word suffer. No image. No symbols. No meaning. No Gods: No Religion.

For is it not the empty hand, and the empty hand alone, that can be filled? As long as we cling to our religious traditions, we pretend to be in possession of something. We thereby prevent the advent of what can come, if at all, only as the free gift of the real world to him who is ready to receive because he has nothing whatsoever of his own accord, as the gift to him who no longer, with a modesty that is disguised arrogance, denounces our poverty as nihilism, but comprehends it as the presence of the unknown future.[9]

[9] Giegerich, "Rupture, or: Psychology and Religion," *CEP*, Vol I, p. 231.

Part Three

> I only know—and here I am expressing what countless other people know—that the present is a time of God's death and disappearance. The myth says he was not to be found where his body was laid. "Body" means the outward, visible form, the erstwhile but ephemeral setting for the highest value. The myth further says that the value rose again in a miraculous manner, transformed. It looks like a miracle, for, when a value disappears, it always seems to be lost irretrievably. So it is quite unexpected that it should come back. The three days' descent into hell during death describes the sinking of the vanished value into the unconscious, where, by conquering the power of darkness, it establishes a new order, and then rises up to heaven again, that is, attains supreme clarity of consciousness. The fact that only a few people see the Risen One means that no small difficulties stand in the way of finding and recognizing the transformed value.
>
> C. G. Jung (*CW* 11 § 149)

The God-Question Again

For the sake of completeness we should probably take another look at the question we began with— "Do you believe in God?"—examining it in the light of the analytic attitude that Giegerich has distilled from Jung's psychology via the process of immanent critique.

The first step in this effort requires the setting aside of a bias of Jung's that led him to regard this question as being psychologically irrelevant. I refer here to Jung's privileging of an empirical approach over a speculative one. In default of his own recognition that the psyche is at once its own subject and object (a recognition that simply requires a speculative approach), Jung set himself up as an empiricist observing the facts of the psychic process. It was as if he had said, forget about the invisible, intangible, (and yet!) intelligible forest, forget about the invisible, intangible, and yet intelligible soul, just look at all the trees, or in Jung's case, all the God-images.

Consider for example his rejoinder to H. L. Philp. After reminding Jung of his statement in *Answer to Job*, "God is an obvious psychic and non-physical fact," Philp had added, "But I feel in the end you do not actually answer the question as to whether or not you believe in the existence of God other than as an archetype. Do you?" Answering at length Jung first discusses epistemological issues he was mindful of in formulating his archetype concept and then, speaking more directly to the question Philp had put, avers that:

> Speaking for myself, the question whether God exists or not is futile. I am sufficiently convinced of the effects man has always attributed to a divine being. If I should express a belief beyond that or should assert the existence of God, it would not only be superfluous and inefficient, it would show that I am not basing my opinion on facts. When people say they believe in the existence of God, it has never impressed me in the least. Either I know a thing and then I don't need to believe it; or I believe it because I am not sure that I know it. I am well satisfied with the fact that I know experiences which I cannot avoid calling numinous or divine. (*CW* 18 § 1589)

This is a tricky passage. On the surface of it, at least, the distinction between knowing and believing makes a lot of sense and we readily accept the image it suggests to us of Jung as a responsible and circumspect scientist. But this is only how it appears on the surface. Reading between the lines we find that they also comprise a diminutive version of the emphatic assertion that he would later make in his interview with the BBC, "I *know*. I don't need to believe. I know."[1] I say "diminutive version" here because in the BBC interview Jung claims to know God, while in the more considered passage that we are now examining it is "*experiences*" that he knows, "experiences which [he] cannot avoid calling numinous or divine." We may be reminded by this of yet another passage that we discussed earlier, the one in which Jung declared, "Religious experience is absolute; it cannot be disputed" (*CW* 11 § 167). Jung, I submit, is having much the same conversation with his theological critic Philp as he presented in that earlier text: "You can only say that you have never had such an experience, whereupon your opponent will reply: 'Sorry, I have.' And there your discussion will come to an end" (*CW* 11 § 167).

But are the soul and its highest value, God, something that we experience? Has not our consciousness of consciousness (one corollary of which is Jung's psychology-constituting insight into the lack of an Archimedean point) negated and sublated our relation to what Jung continued to give out as immediate experience, numinous and divine?

In a recent interview, Giegerich provides an important clarification with respect to this question. Asked by his interlocutor to provide an example from his own or someone else's experience of what he means by the soul's logical life, Giegerich replies:

> I am taken a little by surprise by your question. I have to think a bit. I wonder, is "soul" really something that we experience? I don't think so. It is accessible only on reflection and to our insight (after the fact), and this insight presupposes both some effort (study, so-called "analysis," "seeing through") and a particular eye for things psychological. Experiences are immediate and subjective. But "the soul" is, according to Jung [and here he is again citing Jung against Jung—G.M.], precisely non-ego, an objective psyche. He spoke of background processes, just as Hillman located the soul, metaphorically speaking, in the underworld. "Soul" is certainly not about us and what we feel or think. There is no direct access to it. If one

---

[1] BBC Television, "Face to Face," broadcast October 22, 1959. In William McGuire & R. F. C. Hull, eds., *C. G. Jung Speaking: Interviews and Encounters*, (Princeton: Princeton University Press, 1977), p. 428.

> wants to learn something about the soul and its logical life it is far better to turn away from us people and instead turn to myth, theology, archaic ritual (like the Roman Catholic Mass), great literature and art, philosophy, or alchemy, on the one hand, and to the course of real history, social changes, the development of technology and the like, on the other.[2]

Contrary to Jung's view, the criterion Giegerich here lays out identifies the "Do you believe in God?" question to be a worthy and potentially soul-fathoming one. On one hand, and weightily so, it is a piece of theology; on the other, the issue at stake in it has long figured in the course of actual history, real social changes and the like. For, indeed, as we noted in Part One, more blood has been spilled over this question than over any other. And this is to say nothing of the role it has played in literature, art, philosophy and the other genres of soul-searching enquiry mentioned by Giegerich. Surely, then, we should be able to learn something about the soul just by delving into what this question's having arisen says about it. Our challenge, however, further to Giegerich's comment that the soul is not reached immediately, experientially, is to work with it speculatively, that is, via study, analysis, and seeing through.

Speculative Treatment

Approached in this spirit, the main thing to be borne in mind with respect to the "Do you believe in God?" question is that it is *the psychology of the question itself* that we are interested in and not the psychology of the patient or analyst in a personalistic sense. This, of course, is not to neglect the fact that there may be any number of meanings, interests, and anxieties on the ego-level that figure in the posing of the question. The patient, for example, may be wondering if the help he his seeking will be compatible with his religious values. Or, perhaps, the question is indicative of a transference, i.e., of the patient's apperceiving the analyst on the

---

[2] Wolfgang Giegerich, interviewed in Robert & Janis Henderson, *Living with Jung. "Enterviews" with Jungian Analysts*, Vol. 3 (New Orleans, LA: Spring Journal Books, 2010), p. 269.

model of an earlier figure in his life to whose beliefs he was subject. There is also the possibility that he is intimidated by the religious ambience that Jungian psychology, at least in some quarters, gives off and wonders if he is up to this. And in addition to these few possibilities there are probably a whole host of others that might have to be dealt with as part of the routine of analytic work. But for our purposes here it is important to be clear that there is a difference—for Giegerich it is an instance of what he calls "the psychological difference"—between psychology in the sense of the interests, motives, feelings and whatnot of the patient and/or analyst and the soul-bespeaking psychology of the question *per se.*

Jung, of course, also drew this distinction. He tended, however, to miniaturize it in the service of therapeutic ends, as we noted in Part Two. With respect to the present topic, this shows in his contradictorily disdaining the God-question while at the same time amassing whatever experiential, "sorry, I have" evidence he could find to support a God-fearing and spirit-filled attitude on the part of himself, his readers, and his patients. We have only to think of that famously precious statement of his from a letter he wrote in 1945, the one in which he declares that "… the main interest of my work is not concerned with the treatment of neuroses but rather with the approach to the numinous. But the fact is that the approach to the numinous is the real therapy and inasmuch as you attain to the numinous experiences you are released from the curse of pathology."[1]

Now, my point here is not to dispute the possible significance of experiences that come of their own accord with that surplus of importance which Jung, with a nod to Rudolph Otto, called "numinous" (though these, too, may have become routine, the standard fare of a Jungian analysis). Rather, it is to point out that with his assumption that empirical knowledge of spiritual experiences simply trumps the God-question he performs a *petito principii* with respect to it while at the same time failing to consider what the question itself might involve as an utterance of the soul.

[1] *Letters* 1, p. 377 to P. W. Martin, 20 August 1945.

The issue here has to do with Jung's tendency not to sufficiently differentiate the event-character of experience from the interpretation-character of meaning. In Jungian circles one regularly finds that experiences are regarded as bearing soul-meaning simply by virtue of their having a strong intensity. But here I would object that while it was enough for the doubter, Thomas, to put his hand into the wounded side of the resurrected Christ (John 20:24-29), it is not enough for analysands to take their own pulse when dealing with an image. And this is so even when we are dealing with images and affects that have come together to form what has been called "self-validating experience." Having long been aware that all perception is apperception, the question of their interpretation, the question of their truth, is all the more urgent.

We mentioned in passing, in Part Two above, the line from 1 John 4:1 about trying the spirits whether they are of God. There is no getting around this version of the "Do you believe in God?" question. Images and experiences, as self-validating and numinous as they may be, are subject at the same time, in what might be called an animus moment of themselves, to that inquisitional court of the soul which has been irrevocably constituted for us by consciousness having become conscious of itself. And in this connection I am reminded of a statement that Jung made that is corrective of his usual claim that the psyche can be approached in the anima-only manner of the naturalistic observer and empirical scientist. "I see," he wrote to E. A. Bennet, "… that you understand by 'scientific evidence' something like a chemical or physical proof. But what about evidence in a Law Court? The concept of scientific proof is hardly applicable there, and yet the Court knows of evidence which suffices to cut a man's head off, which means a good deal more than the mere universality of a symbol. I think that there is such a thing as 'commensurability of evidence'" (*Letters 2*, p. 567, 11 June, 1960).

This is a crucial point. Immediate psychology—Jung's empirical data of experience—must be reflected into itself via the hermeneutic circle as in a court proceeding or heresy trial, even as in Dostoevsky's novel, *The Brothers Karamazov*, orthodox Christian piety (Alyosha), disavowal of belief in the existence of God and in the immortality of the soul (Ivan), and a murder trial (Dmitry) all figure together while at the same time a story is told wherein the return of the popular miracle-performing, experience-generating Christ is opposed by the Grand Inquisitor for having fallen below the *niveau* of the consciousness that the Church has achieved during the course of its many centuries.

The Rupture in the Question

There are, I am sure, many responses that the "Do you believe in God?" question might inspire, as many as there are analysts and patients. And this is so even if it is not *they* that are our focus, whether individually or as a dyad, but the God-question itself as the pressingly existent expression, when such it is, of what Giegerich has called (with psychology or "the soul" in mind) "the third of the two."[1] Citing with approval Jung's account of his work with Babette and the Solar Phallus Man, Giegerich has pointed out that Jung gave priority, not to the psychology of these patients in a personalistic sense, but to the content of their visions and delusions:

> The attitude of the psychologist is receptivity; the relation into which he is placed is the conversation through which he is addressed and experiences a challenge. That is, the phenomenon does the talking: the phenomenon and not, as one might think at first, the patient. ... What touched Jung ... was the content, the matter, that expressed itself and demanded his (as well as the patient's) attention. And we can probably say that Jung was in general of the opinion that a patient is then, and only then, taken seriously if the *message* that is contained in what he says and the *message* that comes to him through a dream, for example, is taken seriously in *what* it says, in its content and substance.[2]

---

[1] Wolfgang Giegerich, "On the Neurosis of Psychology, or the Third of the Two, in *The Neurosis of Psychology*, *CEP*, Vol. I, pp. 41-67.

[2] Wolfgang Giegerich, "The Provenance of C. G. Jung's Psychological Findings," in *CEP,* Vol. I, p. 137.

Rising to the challenge of being receptive to what the God-question has to say about the soul, perhaps the most important thing to be noted is that the question outstrips itself. I mean by this that as the question it is, it is more complex than either of the one-sided answers that persons operating on the ego-level might want to give to it. This, of course, is not evident at first. Reducing the greatness of the question to the level of our own littleness, we may stand before it as before a mirror expecting to see our piety or atheism reflected therein. But as we have already learned from Giegerich, while psychology can be likened to the reflection in some mirror, its concern is with reflectedness *per se*, consciousness as such, and not with what the mirror is a reflection of. And the same can be said of our question. It is not its answer by you or by me that is revealing of the soul (in this regard Jung was right to be unimpressed by the claims people made concerning their beliefs in the existence of God); it is the fact that it can be asked at all.

This point may be more readily grasped when we realize that it was not always the case, as it seems to be now, that questions come first, their answers to follow. While this, certainly, is how things are for the modern ego, the history of consciousness tells another story. It tells of a time before the asking of questions. Writing with respect to this distinction, Giegerich has aptly described early man as simply starting out with those answers that he knew as his Gods.[3] It was only much later, after much cultural development and at those rupture-points at which the world, as it were, moved out from under the modes of being in it that the Gods had provided for, that the capacity for questioning arose. And so it is that the analyst might wonder: "Is this why the God-question is being brought up in this session? Does its being put to me now announce that my patient is at a similar rupture-point in his own soul's life?

Historically speaking it was especially with the Enlightenment that the questioning of the existence of God became possible. We have only to think of the constraints which Kant's critical philosophy placed upon the knowing of truth and of how this, as Hegel put it (with the imagery of Good Friday in mind), had

---

[3] Giegerich, "The End of Meaning and the Birth of Man," p. 18.

brought the feeling "that God Himself has died."[4] In the case of Kant and others of that time, this feeling led to charges of atheism, on one hand, and, as this was not to their liking, to a flight into piety and faith, on the other. But answers either way fell below the level of the consciousness that was brought by the question. For, indeed, as Giegerich has pointed out in his Rupture essay, "Both the believers or theologians and the critics of religion (such as Voltaire, Marx, Nietzsche) experience religion, logically speaking, on the same level. The only difference is that the ones say Yes to religion and are for it, whereas the others say No to it and are against it. The level of consciousness is the same."[5]

Recognizing in the God-question the implicit form of a consciousness that transcends the alternatives it seems to propose, Hegel hit upon the speculative approach wherein what was predicated of a subject, most importantly of God, was not regarded as its attribute in an external, empirical sense, but as reflecting its essence in such a manner that even if it should be false and contradictory, it would nevertheless lead the mind back, via that feedback process called thinking, to reconsider and perhaps conceptually redefine the subject itself (G = G and –G). It is the same point we made earlier when we said that negation, far from being as untoward and violent as it may seem to the understanding, carries within it the realization that what we had believed to be the case is not truly as we had naively conceived it to be. And it was along these lines that Hegel *thought* the crucifixion drama. "Tarrying with the negative,"[6] even as Christ suffered upon the cross, the feeling that God Himself has died is to be reflected into itself in a God-redefining manner such that what Hegel called "the speculative Good Friday" may earn its name again and again on successive levels of complexity in being shown to have been, even in its darkest hour, as when the veil of the temple was rent and the rocks were split, the first immediacy of what might reasonably be called a dialectical Easter Monday.

---

[4] Cited by Deland S. Anderson in *Hegel's Speculative Good Friday: The Death of God in Philosophical Perspective* (Atlanta, Georgia: Scholars Press, 1996), p. xvi.

[5] Giegerich, "Rupture, or: Psychology and Religion," *CEP*, Vol. I, p. 223.

[6] G. W. F. Hegel, *Phenomenology of Spirit*, tr. A. V. Miller (Oxford: Oxford University Press, 1977), p. 19.

And here again the analyst might wonder: does the God-question as it comes up in this session now carry within it the Passion play of thinking that we have just described? Is the patient now at that rupture-point and juncture at which not he, but that greater subject, i.e., the psychology he exists as, is being led under and across? And the question mark at the end of the query he has put, is this to be read as the cross of a speculative Good Friday?

There is a story by Anatole France that Jung tells in *Symbols of Transformation*. Relevant in our context for the glimpse it affords of how the issues that are at stake in the "Do you believe in God?" question might have been represented within a consciousness that was still so entirely theistic that the prospect of not believing in God could not yet occur for it, the story concerns a pious priest by the name of Abbé Oegger who was vexed by the question of "whether [Judas] was really condemned to everlasting punishment, as the teaching of the Church declares, or whether God pardoned him after all" (*CW* 5 § 41). After much reflection and prayer, Oegger's concerns gave way to a heartening sense of the glory of God. He was relieved and reconciled, for it had become evident to his faith that such was God's mercy that he had indeed pardoned Judas. This, however, was not the end of the story. A subsequent event in the action of Oegger's own life brought out into the open what his religious struggle had been more deeply about. "Not long afterwards," we are told by Jung, "[Oegger] left the Catholic Church and became a Swedenborgian." About this Jung comments: "Now we understand his Judas fantasy: *he was* the Judas who betrayed his Lord. Therefore he had first of all to assure himself of God's mercy in order to play the role of Judas undisturbed" (*CW* 5 § 43).

Doubtless, there is a certain validity to Jung's reading of Oegger's religious crisis. On the face of it, at least, it makes a lot of sense to say that "… the case of Abbé Oegger shows that his doubts and his hopes are only apparently concerned with the historical person of Judas, but in reality revolve round his own personality, which was seeking a way to freedom through the solution of the Judas problem" (*CW* 5 § 44). But then again, upon a second reading, what a let-down! Couched in personalistic, psychodynamic terms, Jung's interpretation amounts to the forfeiture of the kind of insight that his analytical psychology was intended to reach. Consider, by way of contrast, what a wiser Jung wrote in another context: "... [W]e are obliged to reverse our rationalistic causal sequence, and instead of deriving these figures [Christ and Mercurius] from our psychic condition, must derive our psychic conditions from these figures" (*CW* 13 § 299). But here, with regard to the figure of Judas that featured in Oegger's religious struggle, Jung resorted to an utterly reductive approach. Oegger, we are told, is "only apparently" concerned with the fate of Judas, his real concerns being rather with "his own personality." From this it can be seen that it was not only Freud, as Jung charged, who "denies the great [and] blames the petty" (*CW* 10 § 367), but Jung as well. Forgetful of the psychological difference, Jung did not match the level of Oegger's engagement, which was an engagement with God, by holding to the soul-level, but explained Oegger's religious question in terms of Oegger's psychology. We may be reminded in this connection of Jung's regret that his religiously conflicted father, a pastor in the Swiss Reformed Church, "... regarded his suffering as a personal affliction for which you might ask a doctor's advice; he did not see it as the suffering of the Christian in general" (*MDR*, p. 215).[1] Defaulting upon this position, Jung's approach to the Oegger story amounts to a doling out the doctorly advice he so deplored in his father's case, witless it seems that Oegger could readily have served as a model for grappling with one's suffering as the suffering of the Christian in general.

Homo Absconditus and the Call to Truth

So much for Oegger and the naive precursor-form of the God-question. What about today?

I said above that the question outstrips itself. By this I meant that the consciousness that it expresses is more complex than the alternatives it seems to propose. Underscoring this point, it might even be argued that it is not really even a question any more, at least not a question for the soul. This is not to deny that there are believers aplenty. Nor that global-reach religious strife has

---

[1] For Giegerich's discussion of this text see *The Soul's Logical Life*, p. 57.

everywhere become the cost of doing business. All this is true, and I should also not forget to mention the commodified "religious" content of New Age spirituality. But meanwhile and nevertheless, it has become readily apparent that for consciousness-at-large what once had the form of God or gods has now the form of "the subject" and that with this development God is no longer the topic that "he" or "she" had once been.

Now, if this is so, and I think that it is, our question needs updating. This, however, is a somewhat complicated undertaking as it implies a negation. To be fully contemporized, our question must be formulated as a "post-question." I am not suggesting here that we actually indulge in such post-speak. On the contrary, we may drop the term at once. All that is needed is a manner of hearing how the question, hopeful as it may be for an answer, cuts into its own innocence just by being able to be asked at all.

At the end of Part One I spoke of the sheepish feeling that crept over me when, prompted by the "Do you believe in God?" question having been put to me, I thought about "… how halting and complicated my answer has probably become, though it be to a question for which my career as a Jungian analyst had once seemed to provide of itself such a hearty and affirmative answer." But now I see that this feeling can come into its own as the updating of this question. The God-question is a question that wants to question big. And this, its bigness, is of the same kind as Hegel ascribed to philosophy when he defined it as being its own age comprehended in thought. Is this, then, what the God-question is immanently about?

Speculatively reformulated, our question becomes: living as we do in a time for which the death of God has already long become old hat, *what does it mean to be up to the challenge of what the God-question now asks through its no longer being asked at all?*

Two texts of Giegerich's bear upon this contemporary posing of our question. The first of these, from *The Soul's Logical Life*, is cited for the sake of the dialectical reversal that it performs with respect to the figure of the *deus absconditus* and the slogan "God is dead":

> In theology and philosophy (especially in this century), a lot has been said about the *deus absconditus*, the hidden God as opposed to the revealed God. The *ultimate* form of the *deus absconditus*,

> one might say, is the God of whom it has been said, "God is dead." But maybe the *deus absconditus* is more artefact than authentic experience. Maybe the idea of the *deus absconditus* is no more than the mirror image of *homo absconditus*. Maybe this God image is the image in which modern man can know himself, can know his self-definition, the logical status in which he established himself, namely as having in the depths of his Being absconded from the world, even while *apparently* still living in this world. Could it be that "God is dead" is not speaking about God at all, but about man? About *man* being "dead" … because he has forgone his humanness and instead defined himself as a "functionary" in the literal sense, as a functioning machine (even if a very complex one) and because he seems to see his highest purpose in assimilating himself more and more to the machines, robots, and automats that he surrounds himself with? And could it be that "God is dead" is thus not a theoretical insight or thesis, but an involuntary self-expression?[2]

Giegerich's point in this passage is not to overturn the "God is dead" idea. Nor is it part of a strategy to have a God again after all. Rather, it is to highlight the challenge-character of a situation in which "what used to be viewed as some numinous Other has *objectively* been seen through by the soul as a part of its own self-relation" such that "for the modern soul God has become impossible …"[3] Now it is crucial to realize here—and this would amount to the resolution of the *homo absconditus* problem aptly emphasized by Giegerich—that far from indicating that we are bereft of truth, the *deus absconditus* and God is dead ideas reflect a radical form-change in its logic and constitution. Having integrated its former semantic content "God" into its syntax, consciousness is henceforth more explicitly generative with respect to truth. In an earlier and well-known essay, Giegerich has thematized this moment in the soul's logical life as "The End of Meaning and the Birth of Man." The reference is to man having been born out of his mythological mode of being in the world and to the soul's no longer presenting itself to him as divine other. For born man truth is no

---

[2] Giegerich, *The Soul's Logical Life*, p. 227.

[3] Giegerich, in Robert & Janis Henderson, *Living with Jung*, p. 277.

longer received through the immediacy of his immurement in nature and tradition. For his relation to all that is now a broken, reflected one. It has become historical. Nor is it empirically available to him though the supposedly raw, spontaneous experiences coming from *his* inner. For he knows that there is nothing "raw" and "spontaneous," that being only how things had seemed to a more naive consciousness that was not conscious of itself. No, truth now must be generated anew by our coming forward and showing presence even when this means exposing ourselves to the negations that assail us, time and again, at the abyss-edge of the split in the world.

The second text (and we shall be ending with this) speaks to the generative and explicitly soul-*making* character that consciousness, now as *knowing* consciousness, has with respect to the soul and its truths. Drawing upon Jung's statement in *Memories* (*MDR*, p. 325) that "I am *only* that" (a phrase that in Jung's context is used to indicate his awareness that it is only through the embracing and living of our fundamental finiteness that the relation to the infinite is opened up), Giegerich writes:

> When I am "*only* that," I am without higher orders, even without the mythical garment of an endowment (be it by Nature or by the Creator) with the "dignity of man" or "inalienable human rights," these inflated modern ideas. I cannot bask in the shine of an eternal truth, an absolute ideal, or higher values that would be in my possession. No such thing has revealed itself to me and claimed me. And yet, this does by no means mean that "anything goes." [In *The Brothers Karamazov*, Ivan declares that if God is dead everything is permissible.—G.M.] I am not without truth, norms, values. But they, conversely, receive their authority and reality only from *my* being-so and *my* standing up for them. In this sense, they are fundamentally contingent, subjective: human, all-too-human; there is no essential difference to my liking this food or art or music and disliking that. What gives them their objectivity is the objective fact of my being-so. In the "Prologue" to *Memories, Dreams, Reflections* Jung wrote, "Whether or not the stories [that he was going to tell] are 'true' is not the problem. The only problem is whether what I tell is *my* fable, *my* truth." … This is said in the spirit of truly being "*only* that."

Continuing, Giegerich adds,

> Certain things, views, possible behaviours, etc., happen to be incompatible with who and how I am. *This* is the only "proof" I have to offer for my truths. Here I stand, I cannot do otherwise. But here I *do* stand, and really *stand.*

And then there is this:

> In order to find *my* truth and my *truth*, I have to perceive, alchemically speaking, as the *homo totus* and observe, while focussing on the *logos* as the soul of my world, my wholehearted responses.[4]

Jungian analysis *post mortem dei.* The reason for my title is now fully disclosed. Prompted by Giegerich's essay to recall occasions when the God-question has been put to me (while being cognizant at the same time of Jung's characterization of the present as "a time of God's death and disappearance"), I have endeavoured in these pages to work out *my* answer. Coming forward and showing presence after much study, analysis and seeing-through, I can state it now in a line or two: it is only by our *thinking the death of God,* here at the abyss-edge of the split in the world, that the birth of man, and along with this the challenge of *becoming self* (I refer to *psychology's* attaining the form of self in contra-distinction to your or my *having a relationship to the Self* on the model of a relation to God!), truly comes into its own. With Jung, against Jung, beyond Jung, and this in the spirit of being "*only* that": individuation after all.

---

[4] Giegerich, "The End of Meaning and the Birth of Man," p. 32.

Appendix

Guest Editor's Introduction for *Spring Journal's* "Jung and Christianity" Issue[1]

It is Jung's (some might say, dubious) distinction to have developed a psychology "with God" at a time that he himself described as "a time of God's death and disappearance."[2] In this issue of our journal an essay by Wolfgang Giegerich that critically examines this important aspect of Jung's psychology project is examined in its turn by seven invited respondents. Conceived in the spirit of an immanent critique (all of our authors are long-time contributors to Jungian psychology), both Jung's treatment of Christianity and Giegerich's incisive questioning of this are discussed in a manner that dovetails with that recent trend within the broader discourses of philosophy and critical theory which goes by the name of the "theological turn." I refer here to the shift from the linguistic focus of postmodernism in general and deconstruction in particular to a focus upon that subject whose development by means of a succession of God-images, and culminating in the death of God experience of the 19th and 20th centuries, has been constitutive of modern consciousness. This is not to imply that Jung's understanding of the psychology that has come to bear his name was in step with this development. On the contrary, compared to this line of thought his "theological turn," if we may call it that, was a decidedly conservative one. Railing

---

1 Greg Mogenson, "Guest Editor's Introduction," *God Must Not Die! (Or Must He?): Jung and Christianity, Spring: A Journal of Archetype and Culture*, Vol. 84 (Fall 2010), pp. 1-10.

2 C. G. Jung, *CW* 11 § 149.

against what he regarded as the deleterious effect of the rationalistic spirit of his times upon the larger sense of man's soul that had traditionally been mediated by myth and religion, Jung championed the irrational psyche, that age-old storehouse of animating images, as the enduring source of spiritual renewal for our benighted modern age. "We should never identify ourselves with reason," he warned (with the creeping scourge of intellectualism, atheism, secularism, and political totalitarianism in mind), "for man is not and never will be a creation of reason alone …." Reiterating this point, he then reached out beyond the horizon lines which he believed reason to have too narrowly drawn: "The irrational," he declared, "cannot be and must not be extirpated. The gods cannot and must not die."[3]

The last line of this quote is very close to the wording of the title that Giegerich has given to his essay in this volume, "God Must Not Die!," while the earlier one in which we are cautioned against identifying ourselves with reason alone is taken up in its subtitle, "C. G. Jung's Thesis of the One-Sidedness of Christianity." It was Jung's contention that the critical rationalism that had developed within Christianity had gotten so carried away with itself that Western man had landed himself in the predicament that his consciousness was cut off from its life-source in the unconscious. Hoping to remedy this situation, Jung trained his analyst's gaze upon Christianity. Effete though it had become, it was Jung's position that a resurgent version of its life-giving powers was immediately present in the symptomatic suffering of neurotic patients even as what psychoanalysis had conceptualized as "the libido" could be interpreted from above (or from more deeply below) as the vitalizing reappearance of what had formerly been symbolized as the wine of Dionysus and the blood of Christ.

This, at any rate, was the vision of analysis that he proposed in an early letter:

> … [W]e must give [psychoanalysis] time to infiltrate into people from many centers, to revivify among intellectuals a feeling for symbol and myth, ever so gently to transform Christ back into the soothsaying god of the vine, which he was, and in this way

---

[3] Jung, *CW* 7 § 111.

> absorb those ecstatic instinctual forces of Christianity for the one purpose of making the cult and the myth what they once were—a drunken feast of joy where man regained the ethos and holiness of an animal. That was the beauty and purpose of classical religion, which from God knows what temporary biological needs has turned into a Misery Institute. Yet what infinite rapture and wantonness lies dormant in our religion, waiting to be led back to their true destination! A genuine and proper … development ... must … bring to fruition … the agony and ecstasy over the dying and resurgent god, the mythic power of the wine, the awesome anthropophagy of the Last Supper—only this …development can serve the vital forces of religion. (Jung to Freud, Feb. 11, 1910)[4]

Steeped as he was in mythology, Jung modelled his conception of psychoanalysis upon the pattern of its dying and resurgent gods. Just as the resurrected Christ had appeared to the disciples after his death "… that they might have life and have it more abundantly" (John 10:10), so analysis, in Jung's view, had reversed Nietzsche's verdict concerning the death of God through the life-giving God-images from the unconscious that it offered as its sacrament.

But did Jung get this right? Was the death of God in the modern sense that Nietzsche had announced it really nothing more than the latest version of this age-old archetypal pattern? Or did it rather reflect an altogether more decisive change in the life of consciousness: the passing away or going under of the mythic mode of apperception *per se*, of the religious mode of having a God as such—and this, moreover, not as some pathological incursion of dissociated reason upon the soul, but as the soul's own doing, its critical turning upon itself in a syzygial, anima-negating/animus-sublating moment of itself?

In numerous papers written during the last few decades, and again now in his essay for this volume, Giegerich's reading of what he calls "the soul's logical life" has taken this tack. Basing himself upon Jung's account of the death of symbols, Giegerich has reached the conclusion—so very different from Jung's—that

---

[4] C. G. Jung, *Letters, Vol. 1*: 1906-1950, ed. G. Adler and A. Jaffé, tr. R. F. C. Hull (Princeton, N. J.: Princeton University Press, 1975), p. 18.

the death of God, or as this has also been figured, the end of meaning, has had to do with the integration of this great symbol into the *form* of consciousness itself such that man comes fully and self-responsibly into his own *as* man.

The back-story here has to do with Jung's important insight that the life of a symbol resides in its being an "expression for something that cannot be characterized in any other or better way."[5] Likening this to a state of pregnancy, the great psychologist went on to speak in the same breath of its parturition and demise: "The symbol is alive only so long as it is pregnant with meaning. But once its meaning has been born out of it, once that expression is found which formulates the thing sought, expected, or divined even better than the hitherto accepted symbol, then the symbol is *dead*, i.e., it possesses only an historical significance."

Apropos of this development, Giegerich has read "the death of God" as the death of that greatest of all symbols. As for the "better formulation" or "better expression" that has been born from this symbol's death, this for Giegerich corresponds to psychology, which is also to say, to that determination of consciousness that is associated with and constitutive of psychology.

It is a matter of demythologization. Having arisen from the shift from *mythos* to *logos*, psychological consciousness no longer relates to itself in personified form as had formerly been the case with myth and religion. For the God(s) that consciousness, as religious consciousness, had had in front of itself or above itself as its contents have gone under into the universality of its self-acknowledging, self-relating form such that it now exists negatively, as Giegerich has put it, not as consciousness of some numinous being or thing, but as consciousness of consciousness, mindedness *per se*.

Now Jung, it is true, in keeping with his insight concerning the death of symbols, also regarded psychology to have arisen from a process of demythologization.[6] However, gravely concerned about

---

[5] Jung, *CW* 6: 816. Quoted in Giegerich, "The End of Meaning and the Birth of Man," p. 11.

[6] We have only to think of his well-known statement, "Only an unparalleled impoverishment of symbolism could enable us to rediscover the gods as psychic factors, that is, as archetypes of the unconscious." (*CW* 9, i § 50)

the effect upon the soul of its having been turned out of its spiritual home in religion, he assigned psychology the task of continuing the soul's religious life via the analysis of the unconscious. Though God had outwardly died (this seems to have been his view), he could still be accessed as the God-image within.

But is it really the psychologist's job to shore up a symbol against its ruin? In Giegerich's view, Jung's attempt to do just this with respect to God shows him to have been unwilling to follow the soul's own process, at least not when it came to that rupture-point at which consciousness or the soul had turned against its having to have the form of God. This, of course, is a familiar resistance. In his poem, "The World is Too Much with Us," Wordsworth wistfully laments the alienation that modernity has brought and then, in a line that anticipates Jung's effort to carry on what he called "the symbolic life," declares that he'd "rather be / A Pagan suckled in a creed outworn"[7] than give in to modernity, which he feels puts humanity "out of tune" with Nature. But the modern world *is* with us! There is no denying that—at least not credibly. Having emancipated itself from religion, the spirit that "bloweth where it listeth" (John 3:8, KJV) has now transformed itself into money, medial-technology, and cyberspace. Rather than deploring these uncanny phenomena of our modern situation (or seeking refuge from them, as Jung was wont to do, in the 16th century atmosphere of his Bollingen tower[8]), the challenge for the psychologist is simply to discern what they say about consciousness or reveal about the soul.

In numerous books and articles, Giegerich has taken up this challenge. Mindful of Jung's dictum that the doctor must be as much in the analysis as the patient, he has again and again brought analytical psychology before the bar of the phenomena that have concerned it in order to see whether its own constitution as psychology is truly up to or in accord with the interpretations it metes out. Now in his essay for this volume, it is not the aforementioned realities of our modern world—money, medial-

---

[7] William Wordsworth, "The World is Too Much with Us," lines 9-10.

[8] For Giegerich's discussion of this problem, see his "The End of Meaning and the Birth of Man," pp. 47-48. Also, *CEP*, Vol. IV, pp. 262-264.

technology, and cyberspace—that are subjected to this treatment,[9] but the interpretation of Christianity that Jung put forward in an effort to stave these off. Critical of Jung's efforts to therapeutically revivify Christianity, Giegerich points out that the negation of God is inherent in Christianity itself. Long before Nietzsche had announced the death of God, the Christian soul had already (though, of course, only implicitly) emancipated itself from having to have a God through that central, form-changing mystery wherein its incarnate God empties himself of his divinity and dies on the Cross as a man—or so Giegerich contends in the course of showing up what he regards as the errant positivity that Jungian psychology and popular Christianity both share.

These, of course, are contentious claims. In a veritable cascade of powerfully argued papers, and again now in his essay for this volume, Giegerich's Jungian critique of Jung has led him to a very different reading of what Christianity and psychology are about than the one that Jung promoted. The question arises: Does this show, as some of his critics contend, that Giegerich is a contrarian who has gone off on a hobby-horse of his own? Or is it rather the case, as others maintain, that even where Jung's views are contradicted, Giegerich's contribution is to be taken seriously into account as a radical and contemporizing "return to Jung" inasmuch as its insights are the result of a deep fealty to and a thoroughgoing application of essential impulses and interpretive gestures that are at the heart of Jung's own psychological vision?

To help us with this question, responses from upwards of a dozen Jungian writers, many of whom have had a special interest in the topic of Jung and Christianity, were invited. Of course, not everyone that was asked to participate agreed to do so. This, as I was told, had mostly to do with being busy with other projects, the upcoming IAAP conference in Montreal being the most commonly mentioned reason for having to pass on the opportunity. In some cases, however, a particular colleague's decision not to participate seemed to have the quality of a response. There were a few, for example, who after reading Giegerich's essay expressed antipathy towards the project.

---

[9] For Giegerich's analysis of these topics see his *Technology and the Soul*, *CEP*, Vol. II.

Giegerich, I was told in a somewhat reproving manner, is "a mere intellectual who has no understanding of the soul." Others expressed sentiments that were the reverse of this. Having not yet come fully to grips with the daunting challenge which Giegerich's writings pose, one of these said that he did not feel up to the task. Another who admitted to "a testy admiration" of Giegerich said she did not feel she should "punch above [her] weight-class"! So in the end, though I had solicited responses from far and wide, it was mostly long time contributors to *Spring Journal* that accepted my invitation.

The first of these was David Miller. Giegerich had sent his paper to David and me just after it was written. While both of us were struck by its importance, it was David who brought it to Nancy Cater's attention, and she in turn who came up with the idea of building an issue of the journal around it. Written from his background in religious studies, Miller's response contextualizes Giegerich's psychological perspective theologically by showing how it fits with and carries on from various ideas and movements from within early, medieval, modern, and postmodern theology.

Other complementary responses follow Miller's. Drawing upon Giegerich's discussion of the Christian God's emptying himself of his divinity even as he dies on the cross as a man, Michael Whan ventures a new interpretation of Jung's vision of the green-gold Christ as signifying the Holy Spirit's self-iconoclastic release from the imaginal mode of thought to which Jung, regressing behind the *telos* of his own vision, clung. And in an essay that demonstrates an especially keen grasp of Jung's concern for man's spiritual predicament, Giegerich's psychological approach, and of the Christian ideas referred to by both, Marco Heleno Barreto acquaints us with the metaphysical anthropologist and Romantic *Naturphilosoph* in Jung who, forgetful of what Giegerich has called "the psychological difference," time and again transgressed the limits of a rigorously psychological approach. And then there is the essay by John Peck. After reminding us of the event/happening/pure occurrence character of Jung's psychology, Peck examines Giegerich's critique of Jung's formulation of this by reading it in relation to aphorisms of Pascal's having to do with thought as that "double inclusion" wherein the impactful surround of events and happenings are interiorized into themselves.

Less sympathetic with respect to Giegerich's critique of Jung are the contributions of our next two authors, John Haule and Glen Slater. Taking exception to Giegerich's having focused so exclusively upon Jung's *Answer to Job*, Haule reminds us of Jung's early interest in spiritualism, of his work on synchronicity, and of his emphasis upon immediate experience of the God-within, while Slater, for his part, antagonistically inveighs against Giegerich's entire approach to Jung and to psychology as a treacherous "mind-trap" that should be avoided at all costs! And then, in the section "Continuing Controversies," there is the essay by Robert Romanyshyn. Written not as a response to Giegerich's "God Must Not Die!" essay, but as a rebuttal to his earlier *Spring 82* essay, "The Psychologist as Repentance Preacher and Revivalist: Robert Romanyshyn on the Melting of the Polar Ice," Romanyshyn's essay, along with companion pieces by Susan Rowland, Joel Weishaus and David Rosen, are published here for their related interest as critical rejoinders to Giegerich.

The final essay of this collection is an essay of my own, "Jungian Analysis *Post Mortem Dei.*" Drawing upon the understanding of Giegerich's approach that I have gained in the course of many years of reading his texts on an almost daily basis, I have attempted in my response both to contextualize his essay for this volume within a larger appreciation of what he is aiming for in psychology and to provide a bridge from the consulting room into what I consider to be his enormous contribution to analytical psychology through the reflections I offer with respect to occasions when the analyst is asked by a patient that same question that was famously put to Jung: "Do you believe in God?"

But before we turn to Giegerich's essay and to the rejoinders of his respondents, I would like to share what might be characterized as a scholarly fantasy regarding the *place* of this collegial exchange. This has to do with the 1910 letter to Freud that I cited above in which Jung enthusiastically writes of the vitalizing effect that psychoanalysis can have upon Christianity. When asked by one of his pupils to comment on this text some fifty years later, Jung answered with some chagrin,

> Best thanks for the quotation from that accursed correspondence. For me it is an unfortunately inexpungable reminder of the incredible folly that filled the days of my youth. The journey from cloud-cuckoo-land back to reality lasted a long time. In my case Pilgrim's Progress consisted in my having to climb down a thousand ladders until I could reach out my hand to the little clod of earth that I am.[10]

This is an important passage. Though it would be easy to argue that the Jungian movement has actually fulfilled Jung's youthful hopes for a psychoanalysis that would "serve the vital forces of religion" (we have only to think of the popular offerings of Jungian lay societies worldwide and of the company that Jungian psychology keeps with New Age spirituality), Jung here distances and divests himself from his earlier views. But as Giegerich has pointed out, Jung's kenotic claim to have come down from the clouds is belied by his manner of expressing it.

> … [T]he very formulation that Jung uses shows that he has not really come down. Because if one is really down, one cannot reach out one's hand to the little clod of earth that one is, inasmuch as being down means having *comprehended* that one is, and has always been, *just* oneself. As long as I want to reach out my hand to myself, I as the one who reaches his hand out still believe myself to be something else from, and above, the "clod of earth" which I graciously befriend. The idea that I would have to come down and humble myself *is* already presumption, arrogance. The noble attitude of humility is the way in which the simple recognition that in truth I am and have always been down here is kept at bay. There *is* nothing and nobody to whom I could lower myself, because the clod of earth is myself.[11]

Further to the imagery of Jung's that Giegerich here applies to itself in the course of criticizing Jung's claim to have come down fully from the grandiose ideas of his youth, I am put in mind of another image of Jung's from one of his late dreams. Recounted in *Memories, Dreams, Reflections*, this dream is the one in which his father is depicted as a distinguished scholar who is also the

---

[10] Jung, *Letters 1*, p. 18, fn. 8.
[11] Giegerich, "The End of Meaning and the Birth of Man," p. 31.

guardian of a crypt in which the sarcophagi of some famous personages are entombed (*MDR*, pp. 217-220). Upon announcing to Jung that he will now lead him "into the highest presence," the figure of Jung's father immediately kneels down with his forehead to the floor. Following suit, Jung attempts to bow down in like manner. But again, just as Giegerich pointed out in his critique of the coming down from the clouds and reaching out to the clod of earth passage, Jung could not complete this action fully. "For some reason," he writes, "I could not bring my forehead quite down to the floor—there was perhaps a millimeter to spare." (p. 219).

A millimeter to spare! It is just here, in the equivocating gap between forehead and floor, cloud and clod, that my editor's vision locates this collegial exchange. Distributed between thinkers of the same or similar schools, this millimeter might be thought to correspond to what Freud called "the narcissism of small differences." But this would be a superficial view. Jung's imagery, after all, is not "horizontal" and "extensive" in the manner of Freud, but "vertical" and "intensive." And in keeping with this, the differences which the various discussants disclose have more to do with the soul-internal, psychological difference that runs through the discipline they share. When consciousness is conscious of itself, a restless tension, born of its awareness of being discrepant with itself, builds up. As if driven by a millimeter gap that it can never entirely close, thought goes under into new determinations of itself via the negation of its own base. And so it is in the present volume. Heir to the gap between Jung's forehead and the floor, Giegerich and his respondents try again those ladders between cloud-cuckoo-land and the clod of earth, driving Jungian thought into new determinations of itself in the process.

ABOUT THE AUTHOR

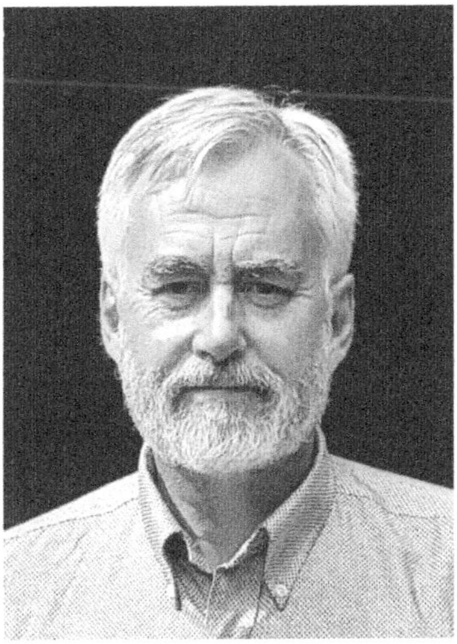

Greg Mogenson is a registered psychotherapist and Jungian psychoanalyst practicing in London, Ontario, Canada. He is a founding member and current Vice-President of The International Society for Psychology as the Discipline of Interiority. The author of numerous articles in the field of analytical psychology, his books include *Psychology's Dream of the Courtroom*; *A Most Accursed Religion: When a Trauma becomes God; Greeting the Angels: An Imaginal View of the Mourning Process*; *The Dove in the Consulting Room: Hysteria and the Anima in Bollas and Jung*; *Northern Gnosis: Thor, Baldr, and the Volsungs in the Thought of Freud and Jung*, and (with W. Giegerich and D. L. Miller) *Dialectics & Analytical Psychology: The El Capitan Canyon Seminar*. He is also the author of three other essays in the ISPDI Monograph Series, *Dereliction of Duty and the Rise of Psychology, as Reflected in the "Case" of Conrad's Lord Jim*; *That Glimpse of Truth for which you had Forgotten to Ask;* and *Inwardizing Rilke's Dog of Divine Inseeing into Itself*.

For further information, visit the website at: www.gregmogenson.com

Made in United States
Orlando, FL
05 November 2026

90230138R00052